MOOD
CRYSTALS

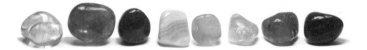

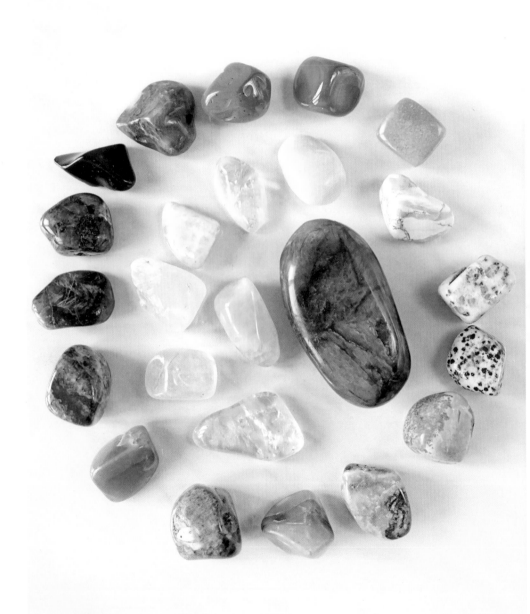

MOOD CRYSTALS

A Hands-on Guide to Managing your Emotional Wellbeing with Crystals

Christel Alberez & Nerissa Alberts

DAVID & CHARLES

www.davidandcharles.com

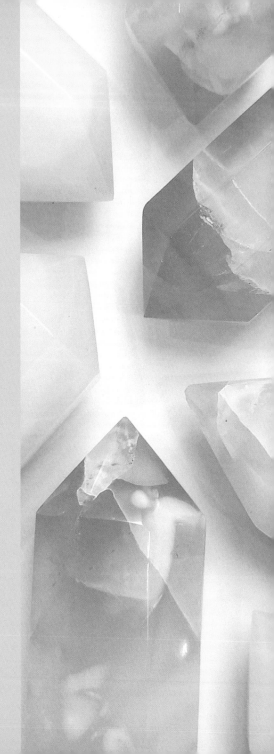

A DAVID AND CHARLES BOOK

David and Charles is an imprint of David and Charles Ltd,
Suite A, Tourism House, Pynes Hill, Exeter, EX2 5WS

Conceived, edited, and designed by Quarto Publishing Plc,
6 Blundell Street, London N7 9BH

First published in the UK and USA in 2021

A catalogue record for this book is available from the
British Library.

ISBN-13: 9781446308530 paperback
ISBN-13: 9781446380420 epub

This book has been printed on paper from approved
suppliers and made from pulp from sustainable sources.

10 9 8 7 6 5 4 3 2 1

David and Charles publishes high-quality books on
a wide range of subjects. For more information visit
www.davidandcharles.com.

Layout of the digital edition of this book may vary
depending on reader hardware and display settings.

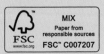

CONTENTS

INTRODUCTION

As human beings, we all experience a myriad of different emotions that have a profound effect on how we live our everyday lives. The awareness of our emotions, or emotional intelligence, is an important skill to cultivate, as it is inevitably connected to personal wellbeing and the vitality of all relationships. Crystals are teachers of frequency and vibration. It is through their specific energetic signatures that we learn how to maintain, enhance, or alter our moods. When we are aware of our current mind state and work consciously with crystals, we can find practical, yet deep, practices to help evolve our emotional wellbeing.

When we first started collecting crystals and minerals, we weren't exactly sure how to use them. We started bringing our stones to the meditation circle we were participating in and began to have these immense shifts and experiences. We really didn't know what we were doing, but intuitively trusted our interactions with the stones. Eventually, we developed a hunger for more knowledge and structure with the stones. One day we walked into a local boutique with a wonderful atmosphere that was filled with vibrant multicultural art from around the world and alluring crystals tucked away in a display case. A beautiful woman greeted us with familiarity, as if we had known her our entire lives. She had an incredible magnetizing ambience about her. She sold us our first pieces of larimar, labradorite, black tourmaline, and a giant hunk of lepidolite, and then pulled out a crystal book we had never seen before. Little did we know, she would be the first to bring many crystal teachers into our lives.

When we embarked on the journey to become clinical Crystal Resonance

Therapists, we had the unique gift of doing the work together and witnessing each other in the process. In those years we were deeply initiated into the realm of working with the crystal and mineral energies. We could have never anticipated the stones would bring up the things they did for us both personally and also in our solid long-term friendship. It was not all rainbows and sunshine! The specific work we were training to facilitate required us both to dig deep and peel back layers of emotional patterns to explore all aspects of ourselves, both conscious and unconscious. Our lives simultaneously started to unravel and transform from the way we once knew them to be. We were faced with the reality of having to create a new way of approaching life, armed with a new perception. Upon our completion of the journey, our teacher shared with us that in over 17 years of teaching we were the first friends to start the training together and complete it remaining friends. It was a true testament to the power of crystals to affect emotional health and wellbeing. We were willing and able, and we valued the crystals as teachers. We allowed these tools of emotional support to teach us to navigate through all the hardships and joys of our inner and outer realities.

When it comes to working with crystals and minerals, you will find that they influence you differently at various times in your life. As you grow and change, so does the energy and connection you will have with the stones. There is a saying, "When the student is ready, the teacher will appear." That has been true for us with all of our crystal teachers, both human and crystal alike. You may not be

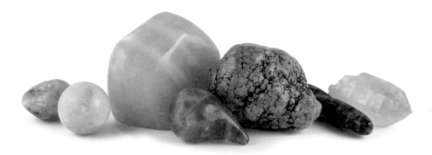

ready for a stone until you are prepared for it. Some stones take longer to work with than others, until they call out for attention. We still have crystals on our shelves that have yet to be worked with!

This book is a springboard, to meet you wherever you currently are. When experiencing intense emotional states, it may be appropriate at times to get assistance in order to discern what is needed. We hope this book is like a balm and it supports you in your journey. And, at the same time, it could give a tiny message or affirm something you already intuit or know. It is an invitation to foster your emotional intelligence and our work invites you to expand your relationship with crystals and minerals beyond what we have channeled here. We all have our own unique healing journey and ultimately it's about

developing a living working relationship with the crystals and minerals to help expand and develop emotional intelligence. Positive emotional health can support or catapult our self-esteem, relationships, careers, and decision-making in a new direction. Emotional health has the power to transform how we experience and navigate the trials and tribulations of life. It also simply makes us better people. We can express our kindness or contribute to our communities and efforts because we have devoted ourselves to self-improvement and self-awareness.

We wish you all the best on your explorations with the crystal and mineral kingdom for emotional wellbeing. We would love to hear your stories. You can connect with us on Instagram @gemstonestories.

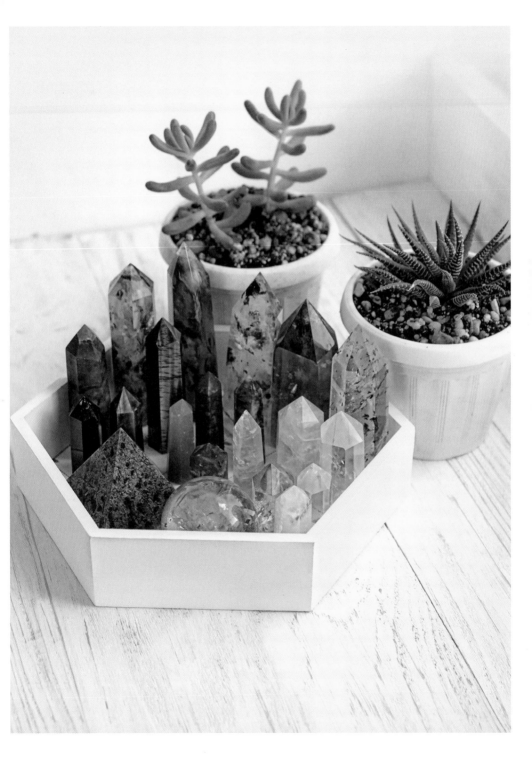

CHAPTER 1

EFFECTIVE CRYSTAL HEALING RELATIONSHIPS

As you embark on the journey of learning and growing with crystals, you may find that the knowledge is endless. If you approach your connection on the surface, you may gain useful but limited insight. If you are willing to invest your time and practice intentionally, there is the opportunity of expansion and likelihood of growth when you truly get to know the stones as individuals.

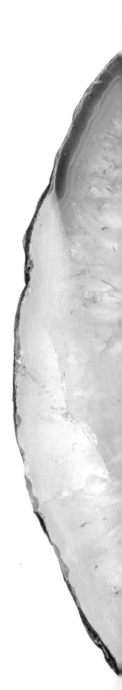

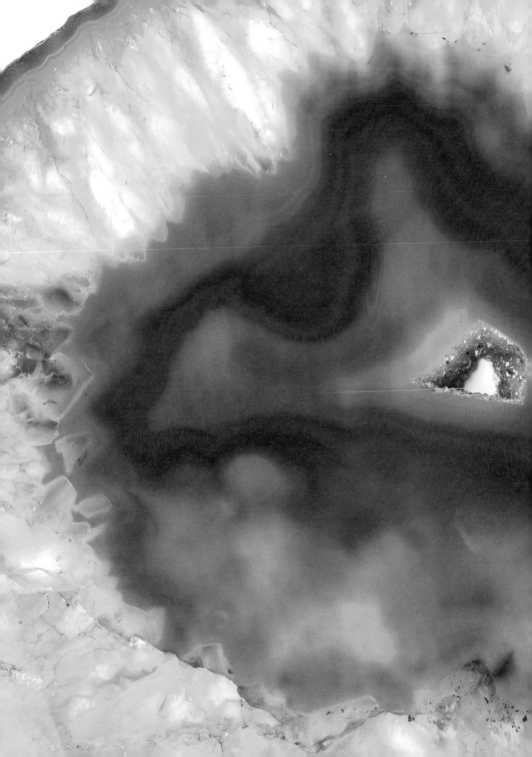

THE POWER
OF CRYSTALS

Many cultures have appreciated the properties of crystals and minerals simply for their beauty and wonder. It comes as no surprise that once you start interacting with them on the most basic level, you become encapsulated by their power. Crystals are here as escorts facilitating a higher knowledge of and connection to our planet.

Humans have a long, rich history with crystals and minerals and they form part of our everyday lives. For example, we use crystals and minerals to adorn ourselves in jewelry, quartz to hold important digital records and programs, and sapphire to make the strong protective screens of cellphones. Our cookware is coated with heat-tolerant kyanite, we season food with halite crystals (rock salt), and copper and gypsum are embedded in the very walls of our homes. Virtually every day we interact knowingly and unknowingly with some form of crystals and minerals. We depend on them for survival, wellbeing, and to maintain our lifestyle.

It is through appreciation and understanding that we can develop a deeper awareness of the potential for profound emotional relationships with crystals and minerals. Humans are redefining the relationship with them to recognize the teachers they have always been.

A self-care tool

Self-care is a vehicle to truly show up in the world and embody emotional wellbeing. It has positive effects both mentally and emotionally, and even trickles further into physical health and wellbeing. Intentional and diligent crystal healing as a form of self-care sets us up for success in overall emotional health and wellbeing. It doesn't mean that we won't experience compromising mental states. Rather, with practice, we can activate awareness and align with the crystals as tools to lovingly deliver ourselves to an emotional state of refuge.

Speaking the same language

Through science there is an understanding that all matter, even if it appears to be solid, is actually vibratory in nature. This means the human body is moving back and forth in motion at all times, as is the crystal on your

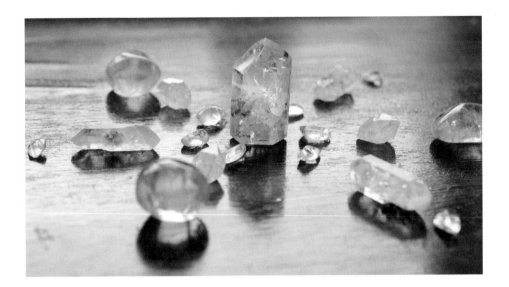

desk. Everything seemingly solid vibrates at various frequencies. The energetic signature emitted by a crystal and the energetic signature from the human body are one and the same—various wavelengths of electromagnetic energy. Essentially, humans speak the same "language" as crystals, from the level of vibration, frequency, and resonance. Crystals and minerals broadcast specific vibrations of energy, and humans are built to process and recognize these crystalline fields of vibratory information. Emotions and feelings are experiences humans have as conscious vibration, which translates into thoughts, ideas, and feelings before it may embody a tangible form. This links the understanding that crystals have archetypal properties that people can agree upon.

For example, during a turbulent time in our longstanding friendship and as crystal practitioners, we have consciously sat and created lepidolite grids to help us navigate disagreements. The strong mineral content of lepidolite evokes a sense of upliftment and cheer. It is through a crystal's energetic signature and chemical makeup that we learn what it feels like to have an abundance of that particular energy. The trilogy of mindfulness, intention, and entrainment of a crystal's energy teaches emotional self-care. The crystals expose us to a strong concentration of specific frequencies found in the earth. Many of the minerals in the stones are also found in the body. Therefore, the physical and energetic bodies will pick up on these powerful vibrations as they have the power to influence our frame of mind. Lepidolite promoted a greater sense of the already joyful feelings between us. The stone gave us direct access to the frequency of positive support to transform us during a time of conflict.

When we are in a positive mood, it is easy to observe how we approach things from a place of the heart. However, when experiencing challenging emotional states, the brain can run away with itself and perpetuate a cycle keeping us stuck in a particular frequency or mood. The crystals are the counselors to recalibrate us back to emotional and mental states of wellbeing, so that we do not go off the deep end and plunge headfirst into an energy-consuming process.

Healing in action

Often healing may be experienced as a change in perspective. In crystal healing, the vibratory nature of the stone opens up a doorway for a shift to occur. Crystals open up access to intuition, and help us to recognize repeated patterns and shift outdated ones. Crystals possess the ability to teach us how to maintain, alter, or enhance emotional states. Before writing this book, we worked intentionally with stibnite for over six months! Our initial intention was to work with it for a few days and then discuss it. But anytime we removed it from our conscious practice, the effects of not having it present became apparent. Our proficiency to complete the projects we were working on, in both our professional and personal lives, would suffer! Our time was not done working intentionally with it.

Stibnite is a very powerful and strong stone of manifestation. Our experience with it was that of putting a dream on the burner and simmering it until it manifests into the dream we were calling into reality. Anytime we removed it before it was done "cooking" with us, things would go haywire! Looking back now over the 12 years we have known or worked with the stone, we see it was always working like that with us. Stibnite just kept meeting us where we were in our own lives and practices. Slowly priming us when we had the courage to put a few dreams on the burner. If we make the choice, crystals fearlessly hold our energetic hands as we entrain to their vibrations and energetic signatures. Essentially, working purposely and intentionally with them may grow you into a better version of yourself.

Crystal combinations

As Crystal Resonance Therapists exploring our gemstone stories together for our professional collaborations, we tend to first work with single crystals as a way to get to know them well vibrationally. Then we incorporate powerful crystal combinations to enhance the experience.

We found that we were having similar experiences working with moonstone together and it summoned up wonderful ideas. One night, one of us felt called to add rose quartz to the conscious dreaming practice (see Conscious Crystal Dreaming). The next morning, during a check-in call together, we were expressing the shared experience of feeling way too much in our heads. We decided to make sure we both added the rose quartz. After intentionally resonating with it for the rest of the week, we both experienced a shift in momentum, our minds became clear, allowing the energy in the heart to be trusted. We were able to act upon some of our ideas a little at a time each day, which had accumulated to be a lot over the course of the week. The rose quartz created a complementary effect on the emotional body, seating us both deeply in our hearts so we could trust and move forward with our ideas.

With consistent and mindful practices with crystals, you will be able to cultivate the ability to align with your desired emotional frequencies. Over time, you will be able to do this with more ease and be able to maintain current emotional states for longer periods of time. As you get more comfortable doing this, you may want to explore the synergy of stone combinations to dial up the intensity.

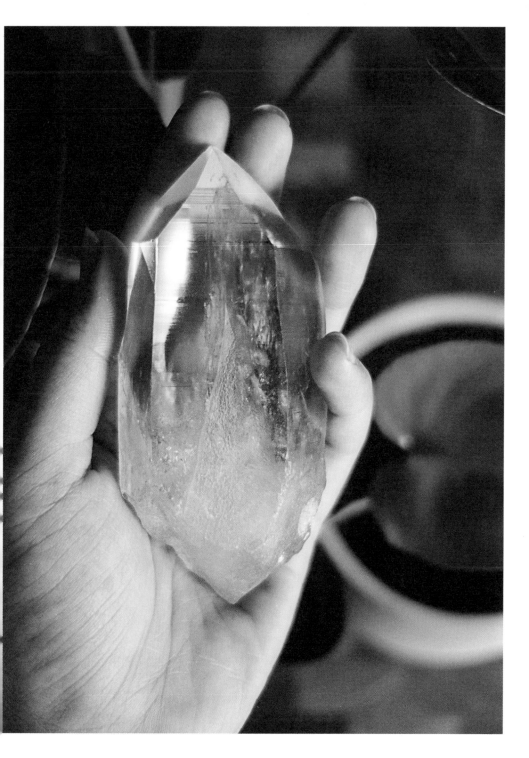

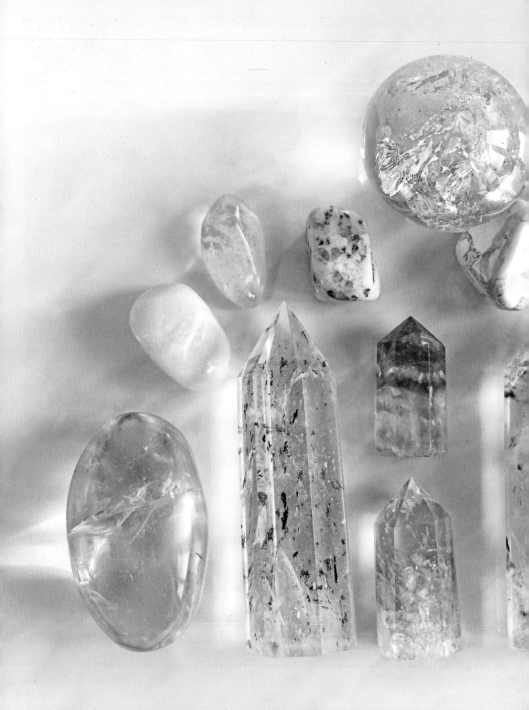

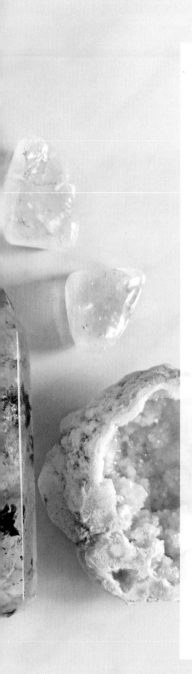

WORKING WITH CRYSTALS

Crystal healing can be subtle or profound; it can come through quickly or take many cycles of sitting with the stone consciously to gain awareness of the way it is working or resonating with you. The information can come through in a variety of different ways and it's not always instant.

More often than not, the conscious crystal meetings with a stone do not produce that much information. Rather, just like exercising, it is the cumulative nature that adds up to deeper and more profound shifts. The subtle shifts cannot be detected if you aren't relaxed enough or ready to see or explore them. Or there may be a flash of an image with an experience with a stone, but no sense of how or why it may be relevant at any given time.

The real gems of the process simply come by sticking to a steady practice. It doesn't have to be a long-style meditation every day. Simply the commitment to engage daily with the crystal or mineral, paired with intermittent check-ins with it throughout the day, are what add up to developing an intimate relationship with any given crystal.

In the next chapter we have provided a series of different practical exercises to encourage you to develop a steady practice.

CHAPTER 2

PRACTICAL EXERCISES TO CONNECT WITH STONES

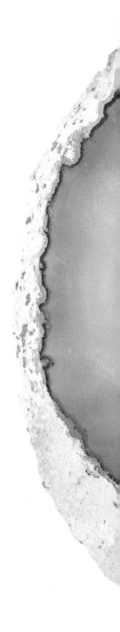

These mindful practices are designed to get you excited about connecting with crystals and serve as a gateway to incorporating them into your everyday life. The exercises will help facilitate a deeper understanding of each crystal's energy, how to collaborate with them to support your mood, personal goals, creations, and dreams, and enhance overall self-care.

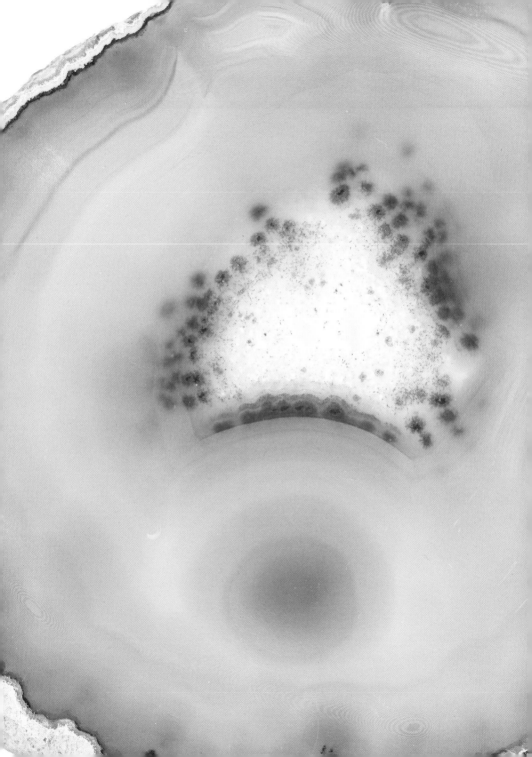

Choosing a stone

Now that you have an understanding of effective crystal healing, it's time to explore the crystal or mineral you are looking to work with.

Sometimes your current emotional state may be quite clear and you will know immediately what emotion you want to examine, and be instinctively drawn to a crystal on that page. However, cultivating emotional intelligence takes practice and awareness and it is normal to want clarity or direction to help you to start. For guidance on identifying your current mood or desired emotional state, use the questionnaire at the end of the book.

Under each crystal entry, you will find a suggested practice you may want to try out with the stone, but feel free to experiment with any of them. They are designed to seamlessly buddy up next to solid routines you may already have established in your everyday life. Use them as tools to help you reset, revive, and reconnect throughout the course of the day. Using these practical exercises as part of your self-care will put you on the right pathway for sustainability and help you foster crystal healing relationships in all areas of your life.

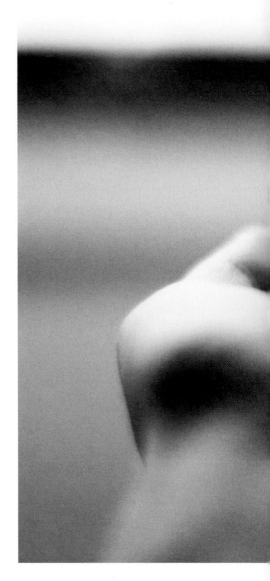

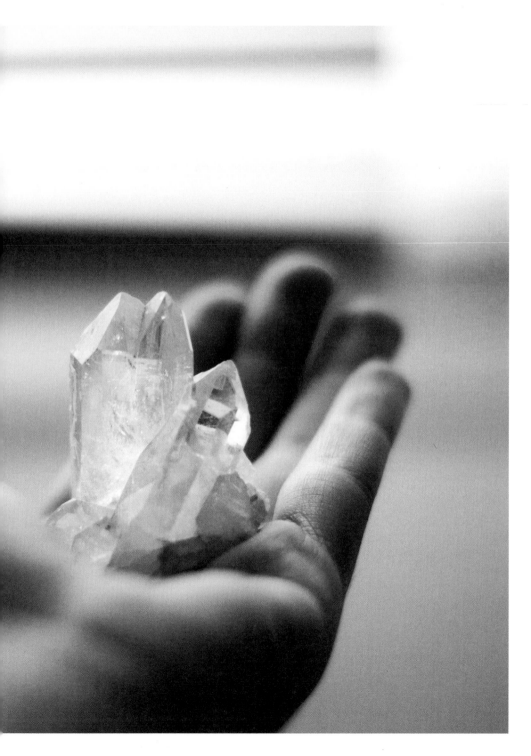

CORE MEDITATION PRACTICE

The purpose of the core meditation is to serve as a sanctuary for the body, mind, and spirit to relax fully so that it can be open, and commune with and receive a stone's frequencies. This meditation connects with the water element as a portal to support emotional and intuitive exploration.

At its very essence, water brings people and communities together, as it deeply cultivates life. Emotionally, water has cleansing abilities to clear and refresh the body and mind.

You can choose to go through the steps of the process on the opposite page yourself or if you prefer a guided journey, opt for the version on the following pages. You could read and record it to play back to yourself or ask someone to read it to you. Or you can find a recorded version on our website (www.gemstonestories.com).

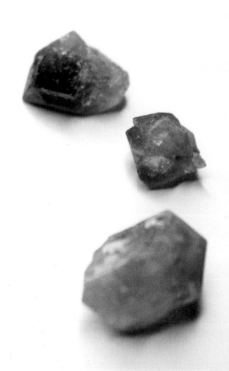

The practice

1. Set up your space. Light a candle, use aromatherapy oils, or engage in a cleansing smoke bath. Develop any association or ritual that helps you to drop into a deep, protected space. Allow your to-do list to be held outside of the space so that you can use this time to dedicate and solely focus on your intention to relax, sit, and connect with your stone.

2. Hold the stone in your hand and place that hand over your heart. As you take several deep breaths, make an intention to open yourself up to receptivity to commune with and receive the messages of the crystal. You can specifically align to an emotional intention or open yourself up to whatever comes through.

3. To begin the meditation, take a few deep breaths and close your eyes. Visualize a landscape near a body of water. Go through the process of physically connecting with the water. In your mind's eye, calmly submerge your body in the water from the soles of your feet, to each energy center as you scan your body all the way up to the throat area. Take a breath in this moment to fully surrender and let go.

4. When you feel ready, visualize yourself safely and fully submerged in the gentle water up to the crown of your head. Imagine this moment of cleansing as a means to access deep tranquility. Then, feel your body's natural buoyancy bring you back up to the surface, with water gently lapping up to the heart line. Let this symbolize the activation of deep listening from the heart.

5. Begin to touch or gently rub the stone in your hand to signal awareness and connection.

Through your breath, sense the essence of the stone begin to gently usher through your being. Spend as much time as you like here.

6. In your mind's eye, when you are ready, visualize yourself walking forward out of the water, crystal in hand, and acknowledgement in your heart for the time spent together communing with the stone. Take several deep inhalations and audibly sigh each exhalation out of your body in all directions. When you are ready to complete the practice, open your eyes and return back to your space.

Take some moments to journal any of your experiences.

- How do you feel right now?
- Did you feel the stone pulsating in a specific area of your body?
- Did you notice any shifts in your being from before and after the practice?
- Did you experience any thoughts, feelings, or sensations?

Record any of the experience, even if it doesn't make sense or feel relevant. These reflections will become valuable to you over the long term of your crystal relationship.

Guided core meditation

Lie down or position yourself in a comfortable seated posture. Grab the crystal you wish to work with and hold it in your hand. Take a few deep breaths in through your nose and expand it out of your body. Allow the breath to fill you. Then on the out-breath relax your jaw and mouth, and close your eyes.

Once you have cycled the breath, take a moment to visualize yourself at a body of water; an ocean, lake, river, stream—any body of water that calls to you. As you walk over to the water's edge, take a moment to take in the environment around you. Is the sun shining? Are there trees and flowers? Can you hear or see other people around you? Are there any animals? As you begin to become aware of your surroundings, take a step into the water. Your feet become covered in the earth and the water. Take a moment to sink into the feeling of being held by the water and the earth.

As you feel into this connection, visualize two cords at the bottom of your feet going down into the earth. Feel how grounded and stable you are. When you're ready, take another step even deeper into the water. Observe the feeling of the cool water over your calves and knees. Take a breath and once again feel the steady energy of the connection the water and the earth are creating together in harmony. Take a breath in here. Pull in the energy and connection to the earth through your feet. Then take another step forward.

As you move deeper, your root and hips connect with the water. Your body starts to become lighter. You can feel the rush of water filling your body. The earth is grounding your energy, while the water is filling you. Breathe this energy into your body. With another breath, step forward to go deeper into the water. The water now covers your belly and upper abdomen. This area of the body is how we digest life. Allow the water to cool the

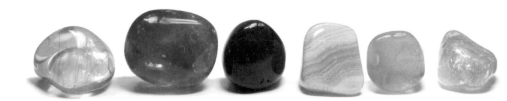

digestion process. Really sink into the idea that the water is cooling and calming you. Breathe deeply.

With your next step, the water begins to fill your heart and chest with the soft energy of love. Allow this love to fill and expand your heart. As you move even deeper into the water, prepare to submerge your throat and head. With a big deep breath, fully let go and sink into the vastness that is life. Allow the water to support you as you float deep into its energy. This is a good time to let go of anything that is no longer serving you in your life.

As you lay fully under the water, check in with your body. Starting at the feet, with your mind's eye check to see if there are any areas of the body that need more attention and care. If so, now is a good time to ask the earth for the energy to fill that space with light. Connect even deeper with your body. Thank your body for being your home. Now, feel the body's

natural buoyancy bring you back up to the surface with water gently lapping up to the heart line. Sense, how the time in the water has created a clean slate and opened up your heart fully.

Now, begin to touch or gently rub the crystal in your hand to signal awareness and connection. Breathe in the stone and spend a few moments of deep listening from the heart. Sense the essence of the stone begin to usher through your being; its energies conversing with you like a dear friend. Then, when you are ready, begin to swim back to the bank and land.

Take your time as you walk one step at a time, connecting with your breath and your feet firmly on the earth again. Take three full breaths in through your nose and audibly sigh them out, directing the exhalation out through your feet. Begin to move your fingers and toes. Slowly, open up your eyes and return back to your protected space.

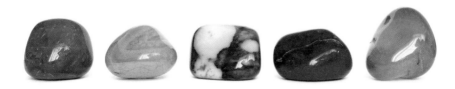

TOUCHSTONE PRACTICE

The purpose of this practice is to get you to interact with your crystal or mineral purposely throughout the day, to strengthen your connection to it and promote the desired emotional frequency you wish to attain. It goes hand in hand with the age-old saying, "stop and smell the roses." Or, in this case, stop and touch your crystal for an express energetic tune-up!

The practice

You can do this while sitting, standing in line, working, or anytime you have a few moments to spare. Hold the stone in your hand with the option to bring your hand over your heart, while inhaling and exhaling deeply. You are simply tuning or checking in with the stone, getting a baseline of its energy. Take note again that this purposeful connection is being established by you with the stone to enhance, maintain, or alter your current emotional state. The crystal's energy becomes more powerful because you are checking in with the energy the stone is offering.

Try this alternative

Lie down somewhere comfortable and connect with your center. Place the stone and your hands on your belly. Track the in-flow and out-flow of breath. Observe how your hands and the stone expand out on each in-flow of breath and in on each out-flow of breath.

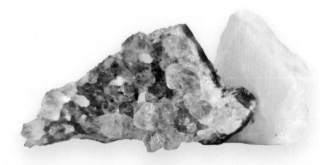

MOVEMENT MEDITATION

Movement naturally creates an energizing opening in the mind, body, and spirit. It gives you the opportunity to connect kinesthetically to a stone and activate a different lens of experience that is rooted in the present moment.

The practice

Bring a crystal or mineral with you to a place, preferably in nature, where you can be barefoot and feel the earth beneath your feet. If you aren't comfortable barefoot, that's okay too. Take some time to connect with your surroundings. Begin by taking a few breaths into your heart and hold the crystal close to your heart.

As you connect with the stone and your heart, and breathe, you begin to feel a deeper connection to the earth. As this connection steadies, take your first step forward. Fully allow yourself space for your foot to move very slowly and touch the earth firmly. Take a moment before your next step forward. Really give yourself the space to feel your feet move mindfully. This practice is about slowing down and connecting with your heart, the stone, and the earth beneath your feet.

As you continue on your path, breathe in your stone and exhale it out of your feet. You may wish to speak to the stone and ask a question. For example: "I am feeling .... How can you help move me into .... (emotional state)?" As you continue, keep coming back to your breath and the feeling of the earth beneath your feet, and allow messages to naturally occur to you.

Try this alternative

This practice is best done while standing. Choose a crystal you would like to play with and bring it close to your heart. Take a few slow, deep breaths into your heart. Breathing into the heart creates an energy circuit that connects you and the stone together.

Once you feel plugged into the stone of choice, put on your favorite song and begin to slowly move your body from side to side. As you begin to move, allow the energy of the stone to move with you. Engage with the stone as if you were dancing with a partner, allowing the movement to organically unfold as your connection to the stone shifts and changes. This practice is all about getting into your body, feeling well there, and being present.

CONSCIOUS CRYSTAL DREAMING

The purpose of this practice is to gather plants to activate the sensory and medicinal qualities of support you associate with dream time. Take time to really enjoy the process of adorning your magical crystal dream bag with your crystal and herbs or other scents of choice.

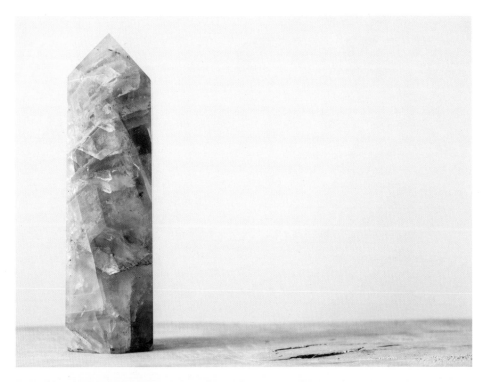

What you need

- Crystal or mineral you desire to work with
- Organza or muslin drawstring bag
- Fresh herbs, flower petals, teabag blend, or loose tea

The practice

1. Before bedtime, connect with your stone of choice. Hold it in your receptive hand. Take a few deep breaths. Ask the stone how it wants to connect with you in your dream state or invite it to connect with you with a specific emotion.

2. Place the stone into the bag with the herbs, flower petals, or tea, and enjoy the esthetic of what you have created with your intention.

3. Place the bag under your pillow (or inside your pillowslip). As you lay your head to sleep, visualize breathing in the energy of the stone into the back of your head. Imagine that energy coming down your neck and shoulders and cascading down into your heart.

4. Continue a few rounds of consciously breathing in your crystal dream bag as you sink further into deep relaxation and rest.

5. When you wake up in the morning and as you rise into your day, take a few moments to consciously reconnect with your crystal dream bag and once again take those first few breaths. Imagine the energy of the stone permeating your head, and moving down to greet the heart. Invite any insights to come to the surface about your dream time with the stone. If nothing arises, simply thank the stone for working with you.

6. Remove the bag from under your pillow or out of your pillowslip. You may wish to take a moment to visualize or manifest the day you want to see unfold for yourself. Hold the bag in your hand and breathe the stone into the entirety of your body. Hold the intention of the emotional state you wish to maintain for your day ahead, and release that energy out of your heart. Visualize this energy streaming throughout your day, touching the places you will go, interactions you will have, or what will occupy your time. Do this for a few cycles of breath until it feels complete.

JOURNALING EXERCISE

Journaling is an effective way to understand your overall relationship with any given crystal teacher over an extended period of time. When you pass milestones in your personal self-care and emotional development, you will be able to see larger patterns of influence the stones had on you during your active engagement with them.

The practice

Invite your crystal to sit and have tea or coffee with you. This is a simple way to incorporate a conscious relationship with your stone and to connect it to something you already do. Having a morning cup of coffee or tea is a wonderful time to slow down and reflect.

Invite your crystal or mineral to sit with you as a welcoming or getting to know you meet and greet. In your journal begin to write a letter to the stone. Ask it any questions you have for it. Tell it a little about what you do know about it or the interactions you have had with it thus far. Finally, close your letter and sign it.

Then write a letter from the perspective of the stone to you. Like sipping on your hot beverage, just allow the responses to the questions to come through. Do not attempt to control or overanalyze it. Simply trust that whatever comes through your pen is what it wants to be conveyed. Again, just like any relationship that you desire to deepen, allow it to be reciprocal and enjoy this way of getting to know each other.

After any practice, you can journal what has come to the surface. Or simply keep a running log of your experiences with each stone and the emotional state you are working with it. You may choose to track whatever feels relevant or comes up. Do not limit yourself. This record will serve to show you cumulative patterns with your crystals over time, so enjoy the process of record-keeping!

SOUND AND STONE PRACTICE

This practice is a wonderful way to bathe the body and energy field in an energetic sound bath to call upon the mood you are looking to move into alignment with. You will utilize vocal toning with the intention to connect with the emotional state you wish to invoke. Vocal toning is when you produce organic elongated sound with your voice.

The practice

Close your eyes and find a comfortable place to settle into. You may be seated, standing, or lying down. Hold your crystal in your hand and mentally invoke the emotional state you wish to experience with the help of the stone. Hold this intention in your being. When you are ready, inhale a deep breath and then turn the exhalation into any organic sound as a way to conjure the mood you wish to currently shift into, enhance, or maintain. Do this for several cycles of breath until it feels complete. Observe how you feel afterward. If you are feeling particularly shy or self-conscious about what you sound like, turn on some loud music. This will help you produce the sound uninhibited and truly let yourself go in the moment.

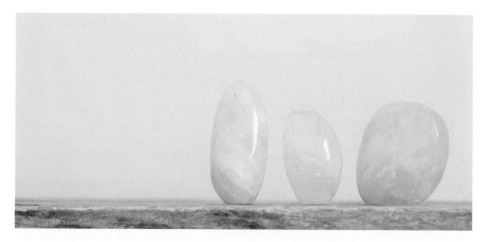

CHAPTER 3

CRYSTALS FOR PHYSICAL EMOTIONS

This chapter identifies emotions associated with the more physical aspects of the body. It describes 14 different emotional states that could be experienced, and a suggested practical ritual to engage with your crystals.

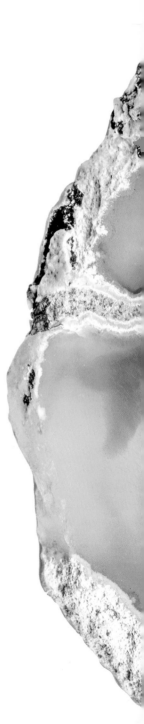

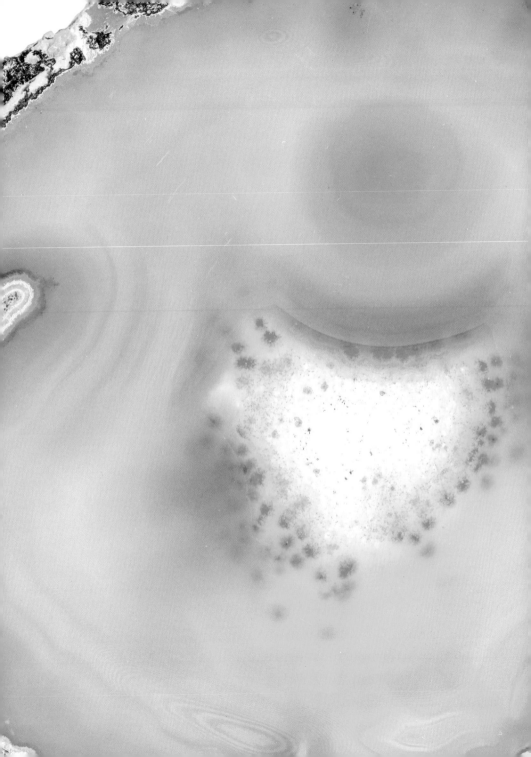

TRUSTING

Trust is the cornerstone of human connection and relationships, and our initial understanding of it comes from an instinctual, infinite place of knowing. When trust is established, it becomes the internal compass to navigate through important moments or decisions. Cultivating trust within ourselves helps us discern what our instincts and intuition are telling us.

Pyrite

Pyrite acts like a building block of trust. Its grounding ability offers a foundation to practice self-reliance. When engaging with the energy of pyrite, it creates a safe container and feeds confidence in your inner knowing and the ability to trust yourself. Its reflective nature reminds you to stand strong and trust the process.
Try this: Core Meditation Practice

Galena

Galena is a stone of security. Its weighted structure protects the emotional body, creating a force field of trust you can deeply lean into. Within this cocoon of safety, you have permission to feel vulnerable in the places where you are still cultivating trust.
Try this: Conscious Crystal Dreaming

Copper

The supportive strength of copper facilitates building a healthier relationship with leadership and encourages a "working together" mentality. It teaches the delicate dance between nobility and humility, so you come from a balanced and grounded place, like a conduit, encouraging sacred service to flow through you.
Try this: Movement Meditation

Green Tourmaline

Green Tourmaline opens the gateways to the heart that may have been restricted due to dishonesty. It brings solace to those spaces still tender from old wounds of mistrust.
Try this: Touchstone Practice

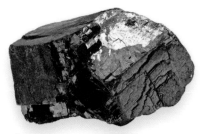

Galena

Powerful Stone Combinations	Pyrite + Galena + Copper Copper + Hematite Green Tourmaline + Black Tourmaline

MORE
CRYSTALS
TO TRY

Black
Tourmaline

Hematite

Spessartine
Garnet

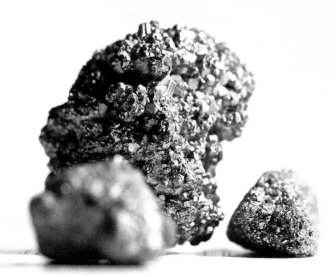

Pyrite has the ability to safeguard
you from potentially destructive
behaviors. Its energy acts as fuel
to fire up motivations and positive
attitudes so that you may approach
life with certainty.

STRONG

True strength comes from a place of emotional intelligence, which allows us to find value in our experiences. The ability to navigate with clarity, tolerance, and a greater understanding builds emotional strength and resilience. Being emotionally strong comes from a willingness to be seen in all forms of vulnerability.

Emerald

Emerald is the sounding horn calling all your fragmented pieces back to wholeness. It creates a safe container to land in and gather yourself emotionally. This stone teaches resilience, encouraging you to get back on the horse and try again. It helps you to stay adaptable in different situations and circumstances.
Try this: Sound and Stone Practice

Diamond

An undeniably attention-grabbing stone, the way a faceted diamond encapsulates light and reflects it out in such radiance attests to its ability to encourage you to do the same. Diamond is like a spotlight to enhance what is already deep within and rising to the surface to be seen. It's a great companion to commemorate strength when celebrating an accomplishment.
Try this: Journaling Exercise

Sapphire

Sapphire nurtures communication when you have difficulty expressing yourself. It dispels anxiety, grounds thoughts and ideas, and initiates pathways to encourage you out of depression or dissociation. It allows vulnerability to come through the surface and emotion to flow freely. When you feel strong, this stone feeds that emotional strength.
Try this: Movement Meditation

Obsidian

Obsidian provides stability and protection, so it fortifies your strength. It can cut through emotional turmoil and provide a safe perspective to look at difficult situations. It can help you recover from circumstances that have disempowered you. Obsidian allows the mind to feel at ease so you may move forward with less rigidity and tension.
Try this: Core Meditation Practice

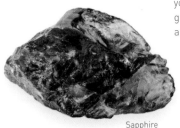

Sapphire

Powerful Stone Combinations	Ruby + Sapphire
	Diamond + Emerald
	Turquoise + Obsidian

MORE
CRYSTALS
TO TRY

Turquoise

Seraphinite

Ruby

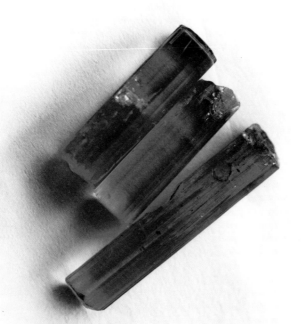

Emerald tenderly mends the feelings of a broken heart. It opens the channels of the heart and fortifies it with the strength of compassion and understanding.

WORTHY

At the surface level, being given recognition brings a feeling of worthiness. Delving deeper, worth is tethered to how well we treat or think about ourselves. When we value ourselves and act in accordance with those beliefs, it gives us a sense of purpose and belonging.

Blue/Green Tourmaline

This stone is an accelerator to the heart, expanding a feeling of self-worth in all directions and teaching self-love and devotion. It redirects you when you are triggered into a low mood or gives you a more heart-centered perspective. It reminds you to speak to yourself as you would a child, with a kind of gentle patience and unconditional love.
Try this: Core Meditation Practice

Emerald

Emerald guides you to self-respect and inspires the feelings "I am enough." It humbly shows you to honor uniqueness and embody the totality of the value you bring to relationships, teaching the concept of giving without expectation of receiving anything in return.
Try this: Conscious Crystal Dreaming

Lepidolite

Lepidolite is a strong emotional peacemaker. It is effective at gently dissolving negative self-talk and opens the channels to surrender into relaxation. It caresses the exposed edges of a wounded heart and teaches you how to mother yourself with loving kindness.
Try this: Sound and Stone Practice

Larimar

Larimar opens the heart to self-acceptance and encourages you to examine if your current beliefs are in alignment with your self-worth. Larimar can burn away the falseness of self-doubt and be the balm to restore an updated reality on your true value.
Try this: Touchstone Practice

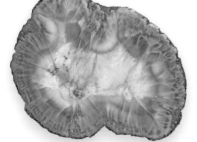

Larimar

Powerful Stone Combinations	Ruby + Zoisite
	Blue/Green Tourmaline + Lepidolite
	Larimar + Lepidolite

Blue/Green Tourmaline acts as a luminary inspiring you to come from a place of nobility. It supports you to trust your value and the unique gifts you bring to the world.

MORE
CRYSTALS
TO TRY

Spirit Quartz

Ruby

Lapis Lazuli (no crystal structure)

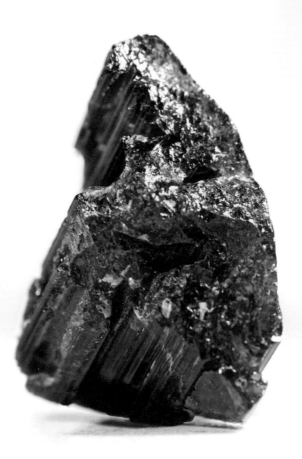

CALM

Being calm is an emotional state that brings peacefulness, creating a feeling of ease and connection in the body and mind. Calmness has a heart-centered quality, allowing us to act with clarity and increased patience, and experience relaxation. Crystals that teach calmness generally have an overall soothing effect.

Kunzite

Hiddenite

Aquamarine

Rose Quartz

Rose Quartz relaxes the body and mind into the tranquility of the heart. Its energetic signature is like a mighty waterfall of unconditional love filling your inner cup with renewed vitality and wholeness. It soothes a hot temper, relieves tension in the body, and over time teaches tolerance for things that may have triggered you in the past.
Try this: Core Meditation Practice

Rose Quartz

Larimar

Larimar has the ability to take a fiery situation and caress it into the gentle waters of calmness. It softens the hard edges of anger and teaches you how to overcome self-sabotaging behaviors.
Try this: Touchstone Practice

Lepidolite

Lepidolite calms emotionally charged situations acting as a buffer or liaison between two parties. Its frequency gracefully casts a mellow mood and a feeling of being calm, cool, and collected. It softens external stimuli so you can gain clarity and hear what is in your heart.
Try this: Journaling Exercise

Watermelon Tourmaline

The energy of Watermelon Tourmaline instantly scoops you up and calms you down. It centers and activates you into present-moment awareness. At the same time it embodies the childlike energy of being carefree and joyful, giving you permission to be in the tranquility of sweet innocence.
Try this: Sound and Stone Practice

Powerful Stone Combinations | Rose Quartz + Larimar
Lepidolite + Watermelon Tourmaline

PLAYFUL

When we are playful, we are transported to a place where we are free to be our authentic self. We rarely forget a jovial person or a lesson learned in a playful manner. Infusing a sense of fun-spiritedness keeps us fluid, inviting a willingness to learn, and an innocence and teachability that encourages growth.

Carnelian

Carnelian conjures up a natural curiosity, like a child discovering the world. It fires you up to create and take part in your own amusement. In its playfulness, Carnelian has the ability to uncover what is at the surface and wants to be expressed more fully. Carnelian encourages you to release inhibitions that hold you back from embodying your true, confident, authentic self.
Try this: Touchstone Practice

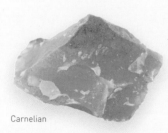

Carnelian

Faden Quartz

Faden Quartz embodies playfulness. When holding two pieces near each other you can sense the energetic attraction, like a magnet. This interaction is like a bridge that releases restrictions and facilitates movement toward connection. Its dynamic alluring energy helps you awaken all aspects of yourself into delightful bliss.
Try this: Conscious Crystal Dreaming

Green Calcite

With its deep restorative nature, this stone asks you to leave your ego at the door. It brings a return to innocence and self-discovery, highlighting the simple joys and love for life.
Try this: Journaling Exercise

Lemurian Seed Crystal

Lemurian Seed Crystal invites you to the land of imagination where anything is possible, activating the visionary and cultivating the inner creator. Like a magic wand, it helps you project, envision, and weave into being what you wish to create. It gives birth to new ideas, dreams, and inspiration, and helps restore hopefulness.
Try this: Movement Meditation

Powerful Stone Combinations

Lemurian Seed Crystal + Selenite
Faden Quartz + Labradorite
Green Calcite + Carnelian

OPTIMISTIC

Optimism is the parent of playfulness—its power is infectious as it sprinkles joy on circumstances or situations. It increases the probability of experiencing success and moving through life's obstacles and is the seed to manifestation, which helps to co-create and shape reality.

Fluorite

Fluorite informs and guides through clarity and insight. It ignites your imagination to reveal what is needed for something to flourish. It reminds you not to look outside of yourself, as the solutions lie within, and it helps you remain assured of your capabilities.
Try this: Sound and Stone Practice

Kyanite

Kyanite connects you to abundance, new ideas, and life purpose. It is a meeting place for your dreams to interact and come alive. It acts as gatekeeper to a clear bridge to move forward, illuminating pathways and reminding you to celebrate the journey.
Try this: Core Meditation Practice

Sunstone

Sunstone helps connect you to personal power, inner strength, and radiance. It parts the clouds and shines light to ignite new opportunities. Its frequency stimulates action and generates affirmations of the things you are dreaming of.
Try this: Movement Meditation

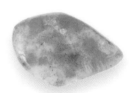
Sunstone

Amazonite

Amazonite clears out toxic energy, letting renewed life trickle in. In loss, it gives you a place to celebrate from in honor of what you are letting go. When you are in a place of allowing, this stone helps give the validation you may need to keep feeling empowered.
Try this: Touchstone Practice

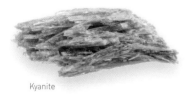
Kyanite

Powerful Stone Combinations

Kyanite + Fluorite
Kyanite + Stibnite
Sunstone + Golden Apatite

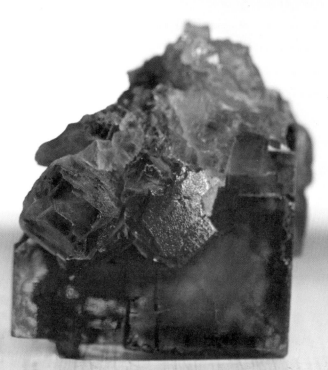

MORE
CRYSTALS
TO TRY

Stibnite

Agate

Golden Apatite

Fluorite has the ability to clear the mind of stress in order to optimize your precious time and energy. It provides a laser beam of focus on your goals or intentions.

ACCEPTING

Acceptance is the state of being fully aware of a situation or circumstance without trying to control, judge, or change it. Emotional acceptance is a cornerstone to redirect our energy and resources into a productive path. Helpful crystals for acceptance expand the ability to practice non-attachment and make peace with what is happening.

Amethyst

Amethyst is an intuitive guide that facilitates a deeper understanding and connection to yourself and humanity. It is well known, received, and adored by all who see, wear, or touch it and offers common ground and mediation to all in conflict or opposition.
Try this: Conscious Crystal Dreaming

Hiddenite

Hiddenite helps you to get out of your own way! It shows where in life you are not practicing acceptance, and brings to light the concept of practicing non-attachment to outcomes or situations. This stone helps you to understand that even though something has changed, its essence is still intact.
Try this: Core Meditation Practice

Heliodor

Heliodor illuminates the areas that crave self-acceptance and teaches appreciation for those parts of yourself you may struggle to accept currently. It fosters a healthy environment in the heart and builds further ease of acceptance. This stone's golden ray emanates the bright light of the golden heart allowing you to become fully open to receiving.
Try this: Journaling Exercise

Kunzite

Kunzite unlatches the heart and teaches you to soften armor that protected your vulnerability and open your heart to new connections. It does not matter where you come from, or what you look like or believe in, simple commonality can be found in the container of acceptance.
Try this: Sound and Stone Practice

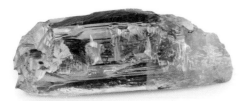

Heliodor

Powerful Stone Combinations	Kunzite + Hiddenite
	Heliodor + Citrine
	Heliodor + Rhodochrosite

MORE
CRYSTALS
TO TRY

Lithium Quartz

Rhodochrosite

Diopside

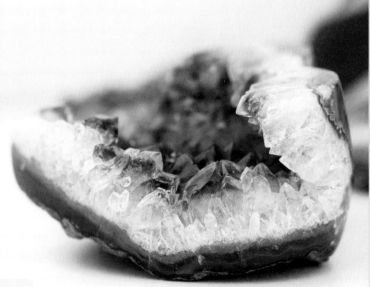

Amethyst is the gatekeeper to
humanity's connection to the
crystal and mineral kingdom. It
is excellent at helping to facilitate
acceptance and understanding
when faced with opposition
or conflict.

BORED

Oftentimes we may feel bored when we are under-stimulated or caught up in the repetitive routines of everyday life. In these cycles, its normal to feel a loss of connection to creativity or the sources that feed passion into life. With change on the horizon, we can gain momentum.

MORE
CRYSTALS
TO TRY

Smoky Quartz

Picture Jasper

Iceland Spar
(clear calcite)

Orange Calcite

The cheerful energy Orange Calcite possesses is wonderful at turning energy into action. It has the ability to open receptors in the will center to generate immediate shifts in vitality. Its enthusiasm is infectious and it inspires quickly.
Try this: Movement Meditation

Quartz

Clear Quartz swiftly moves through your emotional landscape to clear away obstructions that get in the way of being productive. It invigorates life back into passions that may have waned and amplifies creative forces.
Try this: Core Meditation Practice

Fluorite

Fluorite acts like a broom to sweep away the sluggish parts of the mind. It's a great teacher to help utilize your precious time wisely. This stone gives insight to your latent desires or hidden talents and sheds light on where to begin encouraging steady progress and efforts toward goals.
Try this: Journaling Exercise

Fulgurite

Fulgurite emanates the energy of its unique creation. Formed, from lightning striking sand, it offers powerful cleansing when you need a critical spark of action. This stone helps you reinvent yourself with its fiercely effective and transmutative qualities. It provides new pathways for inspiration to flow once again.
Try this: Core Meditation Practice

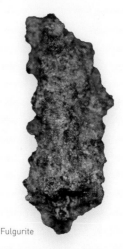

Fulgurite

Powerful Stone Combinations

Fulgurite + Smoky Quartz
Orange Calcite + Iceland Spar
Fluorite + Quartz

WORN OUT

Feeling worn out is the body's wisdom saying, "Pay attention!" It may happen when we are not utilizing our emotional energy well or not listening to our body when we need to rest. Cultivating an awareness of when we are beginning to feel like an emotionally wilted flower is the subtle cue that it's time for some self-care.

MORE CRYSTALS TO TRY

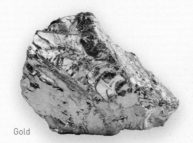

Larimar

Moldavite (no crystal structure)

Tektite (no crystal structure)

Citrine

Citrine gives clarity on where change, or a shift in priorities, is needed. It reveals where a large portion of energy is leaking out, or leading to a worn-out state. Its invigorating qualities can help you feel more energized and lend courage to make changes to reclaim your enthusiasm.
Try this: Sound and Stone Practice

Gold

Gold gives you the energy to persevere and acts as a "pick-me-up," ushering in renewed strength and vitality. It is an amplifying yet grounding vibration, which brings brightness to the depleted parts of the self that need attention.
Try this: Core Meditation Practice

Phenacite

The activating vibration of Phenacite moves in like a summer storm. It clears the slate clean and opens you up to the refreshing spring of receptivity. In this reprieve, you can mindfully select how and with what to fill your inner well.
Try this: Touchstone Meditation

Ruby

Ruby awakens a youthful liveliness that facilitates power and integrity. This stone activates a steady flow of energy, to sustain you and prevent burnout. It lends support to areas within us that may need a little restoration.
Try this: Conscious Crystal Dreaming

Gold

Powerful Stone Combinations

Ruby + Gold
Citrine + Ruby
Gold + Moldavite

FEARFUL

Fear is a primal emotion that humans are programmed with to keep both safe and alive, but it is unique in that it can act as a catalyst or be detrimental depending on the situation and person. Its power instantly consumes the physical body and activates the fight-or-flight response, but it can also have the opposite more paralyzing effect.

Danburite

The frequency of Danburite matches the intensity of fear. Its accelerated lightning-fast energy delivers a crystal-clear channel of acute information to override deeply ingrained programming. In the aftermath, there is a feeling of relief; a ceremonial cleansing, like a breath of fresh air.
Try this: Movement Meditation

Fluorite

Fluorite gives you the courage to examine the root of where a fear is coming from. It has the hidden gift of altering your viewpoint so that you can see safely from a new perspective. Fluorite restructures an overstimulated self and guides you to return to the comfort of strength within.
Try this: Touchstone Practice

Seraphinite

The energy of Seraphinite is one of protectiveness and refuge. It touches edges deep into the unknown parts of yourself and acts like an internal compass to navigate uncharted emotional territory. It has an enchanting effect on areas of constriction as it helps radiate a deeper sense of love for yourself and the collective. It attracts personal healing guides into your awareness, offering additional support.
Try this: Core Meditation Practice

Green Calcite

Green Calcite is calming—its vibration coats over the heart to extinguish fear like a gentle protective shell. It evokes a childlike innocence and restores a natural curiosity about life.
Try this: Journaling Exercise

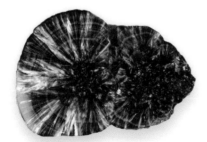

Seraphinite

Powerful Stone Combinations

Green Calcite + Fluorite
Seraphinite + Kyanite + Labradorite

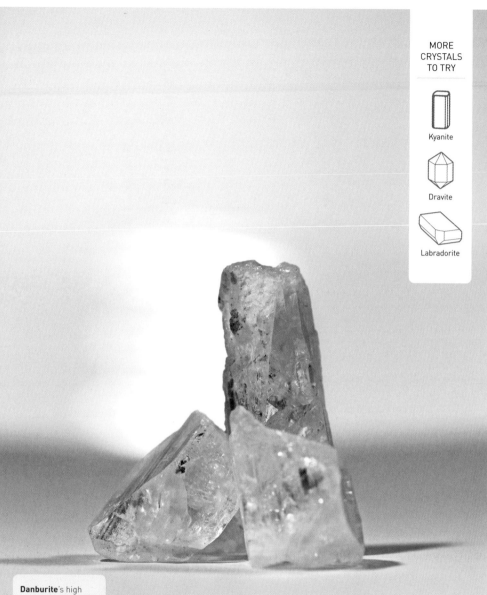

MORE
CRYSTALS
TO TRY

Kyanite

Dravite

Labradorite

Danburite's high vibrational frequency opens the crown of the head, sweeps away fear down through the heart and out of the body and energy field.

LONELY

We may become lonely or self-isolated as a form of protection, or if we are in a relationship that lacks the emotional depth we truly desire. There is a deep longing to be witnessed and cherished for our true selves that lies at the root of loneliness.

MORE
CRYSTALS
TO TRY

Peridot

Cavansite

Aquamarine

Charoite

Charoite clears the emotional state of consciousness to connect with the inner child. It offers a "go-with-the-flow" mentality, giving mobility to feelings of loneliness. It pushes out insecurity and delivers you into the relief of the heart through the breath, nurturing greater awareness.
Try this: Journaling Exercise

Copper

Copper acts as a connective conduit integrating the totality of your being back to life. The grounding quality of this stone helps you see vulnerability as an asset and allows total transparency and self-honesty. It is an energetic, supportive tool that influences you to come out of your protective shell and share more with the world.
Try this: Core Meditation Practice

Elestial Quartz

Elestial Quartz helps you to break free and move out of isolation. It pinpoints the areas within where you may be hiding your light from the world and generates synchronicities that help you attract soulmates.
Try this: Touchstone Practice

Epidote

Epidote offers you the potential to reconnect with life through nature. Outside in a beautiful natural environment, you are never truly alone. This stone acts like a poultice, extracting out the unhappy areas of life and helping you to understand the root of your loneliness.
Try this: Sound and Stone Practice

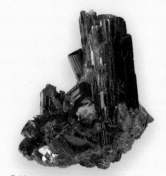
Epidote

Powerful Stone Combinations

Aquamarine + Elestial Quartz
Chariote + Epidote

PAINED

The emotion of pain brings an awareness that something needs attention, or a shift, in order for growth to continue. Often emotional pain can play on a loop that leaves us vulnerable to its consumption. Interrupting the pain cycle allows us to digest and move through emotional pain or heartache.

Hematite

Hematite helps mend and release any trauma that causes you to relive emotional pain. It grants you safe passage through the murky waters with its ability to link the emotional body with the grounding support of the Earth. Hematite's tender approach draws out and isolates the lessons of pain objectively, so that you can embrace what is learned.
Try this: Touchstone Practice

Quartz

Clear Quartz has the ability to bring a clear understanding of the letting-go process in order to facilitate healing. It can serve as a beacon of awareness, shedding light on the places in the emotional body that need acknowldgement in order to be released and healed.
Try this: Core Meditation Practice

Rose Quartz

Rose Quartz can ease emotional pain and create the harmony you need to love yourself. Its vibration can profoundly relax tension in the emotional body. When living in a place of pain, this stone gently reminds you to let go of the burden of worry and helps you to trust in yourself and lean into the loving support it offers.
Try this: Conscious Crystal Dreaming

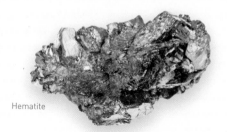

Hematite

Powerful Stone Combinations | Hematite + Rose Quartz
Rose Quartz + Copper

LAZY

Typically, a lack of motivation can cause a feeling of laziness and, if perpetuated, it may unintentionally become a self-sabotaging behavior as the pattern is repeated over and over. Being lazy will suspend action and may cloud our sense of purpose.

Malachite

Malachite's fast-moving energy piques curiosity, gets the blood flowing and the heart pumping, and sparks excitement for life. It adds fuel to creative endeavors to help you ignite passion back into life. This stone recalibrates the areas of the mind that have difficulty following through with goals to fruition and completion.
Try this: Sound and Stone Practice

Epidote

This stone reawakens your connection to the natural circadian rhythms of life. Epidote nurtures you into feeling interconnected with the web of life, encouraging a sense of sacred responsibility. As you come into alignment with the energy of this stone, it opens a deeper awareness of the importance of regular grounding with the Earth.
Try this: Core Meditation Practice

Heliodor

Heliodor provides a charge of exuberance that opens the energy centers of the body to move out blockages that may be holding you back. It creates space by teaching you to let go, take action, and be creative.
Try this: Journaling Exercise

Zincite

When needing an energetic boost, Zincite knows the exact way to energize and help rise up in your power. Its stamina reinforces the tenacity for the adventure of living a full life. This stone's driving force is to motivate you to move forward and remind you to keep taking one step at a time.
Try this: Movement Meditation

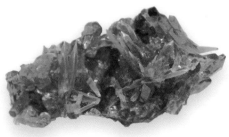

Zincite

| **Powerful Stone Combinations** | Epidote + Herkimer Diamond
Zincite + Clear Quartz
Epidote + Malachite |

MORE
CRYSTALS
TO TRY

Herkimer
Diamond

Wulfenite

Quartz

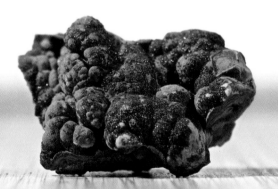

Malachite is a wonderful conduit to spring us into action in life. It moves stagnant energy, negative thinking, and unproductive emotional energy patterns.

DISTRACTED

In today's world, we are inundated with a sensory overload of information and there are many distractions. As a result, our natural circadian rhythm is challenged and it may be difficult to truly be present in ourselves. All too often this perpetuates in us staying busy to avoid dealing with difficult emotions.

Smoky Quartz

Smoky Quartz speaks to the wholeness of your being and carries with it the gift of creating big changes in your internal terrain. This stone promotes strength to root you firmly into your preferred frame of mind and reminds you what it feels like to be at home in the body, heart, and mind.
Try this: Conscious Crystal Dreaming

Shungite

Shungite helps you become captivated by an attention to detail. It has the gift of creating an insulated mental and emotional environment to quiet outside influences or external distractions. Shungite helps put you on a new trajectory, helping you to stay true to the journey toward your goal, free from unhealthy behaviors or distractions.
Try this: Core Meditation Practice

Emerald

Emerald calls your presence and essence back into the body, mind, and spirit. It helps discern where mechanisms of escapism exist and has a profound healing effect on the heart. This stone's frequency provides a blanket of divine love to promote a deeper connection to self.
Try this: Sound and Stone Practice

Copper

Copper acts like a conductor of electricity, giving an inner spark to return to present-moment awareness. Its vortex-like energy awakens the mind to focus on the task at hand and not become distracted.
Try this: Touchstone Practice

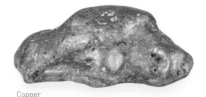

Copper

Powerful Stone Combinations

Smoky Quartz + Copper
Moonstone + Copper
Emerald + Sugilite

Smoky Quartz centers and prevents us from dissociating from ourselves. It brings a sense of renewal and can act as a guide in gracefully moving from one mood to the next.

MORE
CRYSTALS
TO TRY

Sugilite

Tanzanite

Moonstone

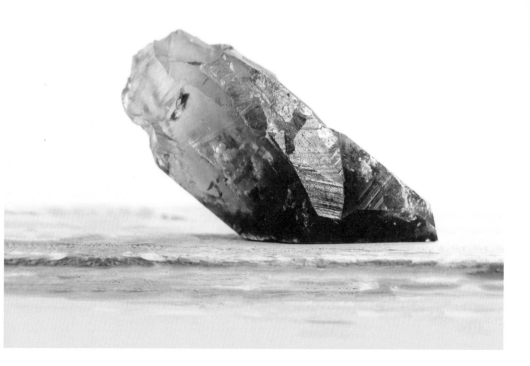

CHAPTER 4

ENERGETIC AND TRANSFORMATIONAL FLOW

This chapter identifies emotions associated with the more energetic and transformational aspects of ourselves. It describes 12 different emotional states, some of which you may seek to amplify, others you may want to ease, with recommended rituals to help you achieve your emotional goals.

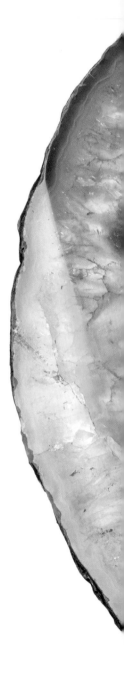

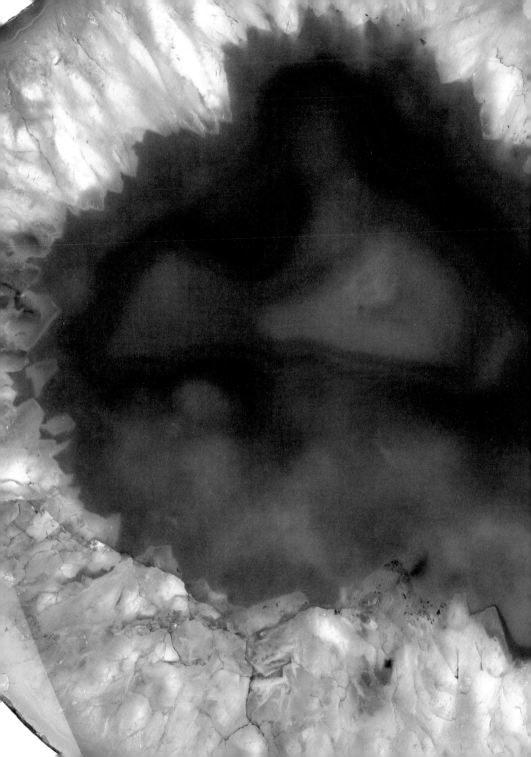

PROUD

Pride is the self-dignified nature of those who are certain of themselves—it is deep-rooted in the heart. However, there is a fine line of duality within pride that asks for deeper awareness. The shadow side of pride can create rigidity, which can keep us from walking the heart's true path.

Citrine

Citrine prompts a fearlessness within to rise up and live in your true potential. It has the ability to invoke passion and creativity into your life pursuits. It is an excellent teacher of manifestation and stimulates the feelings of satisfaction and gratification.
Try this: Touchstone Practice

Sapphire

Sapphire has the ability to ground the physical body and make energy pathways available to flow into a state of balance. This stone can give you the energy needed to move in a new direction and clear obstructions, allowing you to become a conduit of the energy you wish to attract. Sapphire can help to ground potentially inhibiting behaviors into a healthy, humble perspective.
Try this: Core Meditation Practice

Shiva Lingam

Shiva Lingam carries with it an ancient feeling of all that has come before. Its frequency teaches you to appreciate and honor what has brought you to this exact moment. It may be used to move stagnation in the physical and emotional body when you are feeling stuck.
Try this: Movement Meditation

Turquoise

Turquoise has the energy of deep honoring and integration, and the ability to connect you deep into your ancestral line to call on its support. This stone teaches self-respect and appreciation. It helps you find a place of inner humility and balances that with self-encouraging acknowledgment and an appreciation of your own unique journey.
Try this: Journaling Exercise

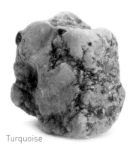
Turquoise

Powerful Stone Combinations	Shiva Lingam + Sapphire
	Tiger's Eye + Turquoise
	Citrine + Sapphire

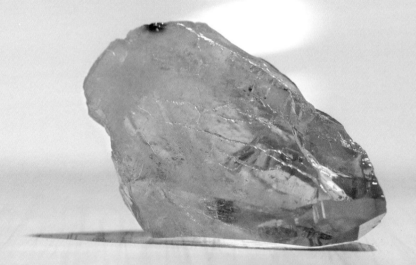

MORE
CRYSTALS
TO TRY

Emerald

Tiger's Eye

Carnelian

Citrine has the power to help us feel well equipped to keep moving forward in the right direction. It is a powerhouse of determination and helps us project with certainty.

CONFIDENT

Confidence is the emotion that points to complete self-trust. It is the belief that our actions will lead to us experiencing some level of success. When we are confident it is easier to accept constructive criticism and use it as a valuable information tool, leading to personal growth.

Ruby

Ruby spirals through you clearing away energetic debris, which may be impeding forward momentum. Ruby's vital energy coats your being with a powerful fertilizer that encourages you to carry yourself with conviction, absolute faith, and confidence.
Try this: Touchstone Practice

Black Tourmaline

Black Tourmaline can transmute negative thinking, and is excellent at teaching how the power of visualization can develop confidence. This stone encourages you to blossom into your true, authentic, confident self. It acts as a supportive companion, helping you to embody new skills by dissolving away what no longer serves your life.
Try this: Conscious Crystal Dreaming

Galena

Galena awakens your power within. It has the ability to ground foresight into action, creating a strong foundation from which you may grow confidently. The supportive vibration of this stone fosters positive self-talk and assurance in your abilities.
Try this: Journaling Exercise

Rainbow Obsidian

Rainbow Obsidian has the capability to cut through the obstacles at the surface in order to move more freely. This stone can help you see through the different layers of the onion and it creates change by making your look at the hidden aspects of yourself that need healing so that you can move forward with confidence.
Try this: Core Meditation Practice

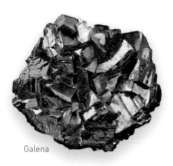

Galena

Powerful Stone Combinations

Ruby + Green Kyanite
Obsidian + Black Tourmaline
Galena + Malachite

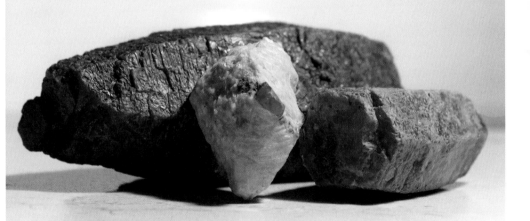

MORE
CRYSTALS
TO TRY

Jade

Malachite

Green Kyanite

Ruby's assertive energy emanates
power and stability. It helps feed
and build our dreams from the firm
base of a healthy, solid foundation.

PASSIONATE

Passion has a direct influence on emotional vitality, teaching us to thrive not survive. It is the green light, affirming that we are on the right track and encouraging us to follow our heart. When we allow passion to organically unfold, we can celebrate the exuberance it brings.

Tangerine Quartz

Tangerine Quartz provides fuel to pour into your passion wholeheartedly. Its high-spirited energy connects you to the inner child, creating a vortex of energy that makes it feel as if time does not exist. It is a stone that allows you to fully be in your bliss and engulfed in passion, with a kind of carefree, joyful innocence.
Try this: Movement Meditation

Carnelian

Carnelian chips away at anything that may be blocking your connection to passion. It helps you find beauty in all the broken parts of the self. At the same time, it can assist you in finding a healthy balance when focusing on a passion without becoming obsessive.
Try this: Sound and Stone Practice

Almandine Garnet

Almandine Garnet helps you overcome an inability to express your passion. Garnet facilitates peacemaking when you are feeling held back from living your passion in some way and encourages you to gently find new ways to express passion to breathe new life into yourself.
Try this: Journaling Exercise

Imperial Topaz

Imperial Topaz welcomes in the rush of energy that motivates you to be passionate about your desires and boosts your ability to dream up what you are yearning to create. This stone helps generate a strong will and consistent effort.
Try this: Conscious Crystal Dreaming

Almandine Garnet

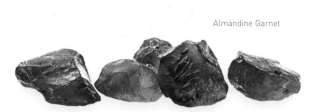

Powerful Stone Combinations | Tangerine Quartz + Carnelian
Imperial Topaz + Vanadinite

MORE
CRYSTALS
TO TRY

Vanadinite

Tiger Iron (layers
of Tiger's Eye,
Hematite, and
Red Jasper)

Brown Opal (no
crystal structure)

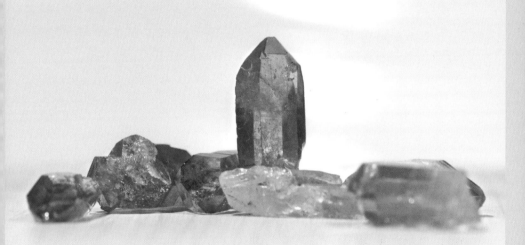

Tangerine Quartz helps heal old
emotional wounds that stem from
misguided judgments from others
that may inhibit us from fully going
after our desires.

SENSUAL

Blue Topaz

Zincite

Blue Calcite

Sensuality is connected to pleasure, the senses, and being in touch with yourself. It invokes beauty, grace, and freedom of expression. Sensual experiences encourage you to slow down, soften, and be giving to yourself. Sensuality may awaken a deeper sense of knowing and asking for what you want.

Rhodochrosite

Rhodochrosite stimulates a willingness to embrace your sensual nature. It teaches body positivity, self-love, and adoration for your sacred vessel. The stone's gentle frequency centers the heart and mind to allow you to relax, with the security of exploring with greater liberation.
Try this: Core Meditation Practice

Orange Kyanite

Orange Kyanite brings playfulness to your sensual nature. It acts as a bridge for self-care and can assist those who have a low sex drive. This stone activates the lower chakra system to energize your sexual expression and enjoyment.
Try this: Movement Meditation

Shiva Lingam

Shiva Lingam encourages sensuality through enjoying your physicality. Its warmth and safety enables you to be protected and yet vulnerable to fully embody sensual practices. It channels the ancient energy of the kundalini snake rising from within, activating the energetic systems of the body.
Try this: Sound and Stone Practice

Fire Opal

Fire Opal encapsulates a sense of euphoria and the exploration of the senses. Its holographic framework and beauty coaxes you out of your protective shell to access your sensual nature. Its frequency is intoxicating to the senses and helps you to become more comfortable with receiving life's pleasures.
Try this: Journaling Exercise

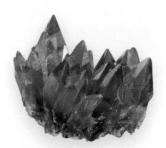

Rhodochrosite

Powerful Stone Combinations

Orange Kyanite + Shiva Lingam
Rhodochrosite + Fire Opal
Blue Calcite + Shiva Lingam

THRILLED

When we are thrilled, there is an intense feeling of being overjoyed. This powerful emotion physically cascades through the body, pushing you to new heights and to learning new things, and promotes creativity and an openness to life. The feeling comes in abundance when achieving a sought-after goal and it inspires others.

MORE
CRYSTALS
TO TRY

Cinnabar

Danburite

Cuprite

Stellar Beam Calcite

Stellar Beam Calcite projects energy, uplifting all things in its path. Its showering effect breeds excitement and it can greatly assist manifestation work, helping to maintain the laser focus necessary to make unseen dreams tangible.
Try this: Core Meditation Practice

Quartz

Clear Quartz captivates all who touch it, enhancing whatever you set out to do through its ability to amplify the energy surrounding it. Like a lightning bolt, it can form a new reality for a current circumstance and make a new path where one could not be seen before.
Try this: Sound and Stone Practice

Diamond

Diamond instantly draws you in and its frequency lends an unstoppable momentum, empowering those who work with it. Diamonds have long become a symbol or rite of passage for people looking to level up and take new thrilling steps forward in life.
Try this: Movement Meditation

Moldavite

Moldavite dismantles conventional rules and opens up a world of infinite possibilities. This stone teaches you to go way beyond the proverbial radar screen and shows you the infinite potential you have access to.
Try this: Journaling Exercise

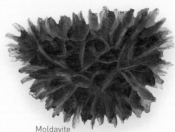
Moldavite

Powerful Stone Combinations

Quartz + Cinnabar
Stellar Beam Calcite + Quartz
Cuprite + Moldavite

COURAGEOUS

When we are courageous, we feel like we can do anything, and it gives us a willingness and drive to stand up for what we want. Being brave is the ability to rise above danger with a strength to overcome it. Courage is a great teacher of facing our fears in order to take a leap of faith.

Copper
Copper's vortex of energy initiates purification of your emotional self. It asks you to abandon preconceived ideas that may hold you back and gives you the courage to trust that the Universe is steering you in the right direction.
Try this: Sound and Stone Practice

Chrysocolla
Chrysocolla reminds you to look within, find your will center, and draw energy into your heart. It opens the heart to grace so you may recognize and cherish inner talents. This stone acts as a direct channel to your inner voice, giving you the courage to express yourself fully.
Try this: Journaling Exercise

Dioptase
Dioptase radiates with perseverance to reinvigorate your overall wellbeing. It serves by filling in any areas of deficiency or depletion within. This stone can recalibrate your mental and emotional landscape when you are feeling defeated and provides you with an enthusiasm to move and grow again.
Try this: Touchstone Practice

Ruby
Ruby helps you face the dangers of self-sabotaging behaviors and transmits potent energy to shift you away from behaviors that are holding you back. This stone's energy surges forward, clearing space within your emotional landscape. In its wake, it acts like a fertilizer to feed what you are seeking to create.
Try this: Conscious Crystal Dreaming

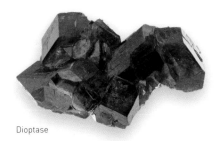

Dioptase

Powerful Stone Combinations	Copper + Chrysocolla
	Copper + Ruby
	Grossular Garnet + Dioptase

MORE
CRYSTALS
TO TRY

Aventurine

Grossular
Garnet

Golden
Labradorite

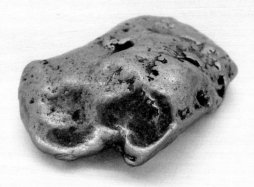

Copper is a powerful conductor
of any crystal energies it is paired
with. It heightens the energetic
effects as it increases the flow of
synchronicity into your life.

ANGRY

Anger is sensitivity's bodyguard. At the root, there is a hidden hurt that causes anger to arise and roar like a lion to protect. If we can find that sensitive place, injustice, or the inner boundary that was crossed, we can find the ability to communicate from a place of the heart.

Black Tourmaline

Black Tourmaline can quickly transmute animosity. Its ability to diffuse and compost chaotic energy anchors you back into the presence of the heart. Black Tourmaline stabilizes unsettled feelings so you can look at them objectively and helps you to connect with the natural frequency of the earth to bring a sense of rebirth.
Try this: Core Meditation Practice

Larimar

Larimar's soothing energy helps to cool down anger and its flare-ups, gently permeating it and sending a pulsation of light into the heart. It creates an entry point and the space to allow the anger to burn off, just enough to open the heart again. This stone facilitates communication to flow from the heart and not the head.
Try this: Touchstone Practice

Kunzite

Kunzite feels like sprinkling a gentle rain to lovingly quell an inflamed emotional state. It quickly improves emotional wellbeing, bringing a clear, calm clarity. It reorganizes the thought processes, especially in the case of "broken record" anger, which can continue long after the initial trigger.
Try this: Movement Meditation

Green Tourmaline

Green Tourmaline is a stone of purity and love. It speaks to the heart, opening the channels of adoration you have for the natural world. Green Tourmaline drops you into the wilderness of the self, so anger is no longer encompassing. A calming, natural remedy, Green Tourmaline offers a reprieve from a volatile state.
Try this: Journaling Exercise

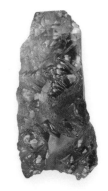

Kunzite

Powerful Stone Combinations	Larimar + Green Tourmaline
	Kunzite + Rose Quartz
	Mahogany Obsidian + Lepidolite

Pink Tourmaline

Obsidian (no
crystal structure)

Lepidolite

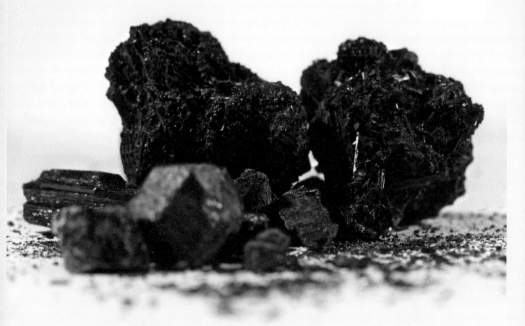

Black Tourmaline extracts anger
and draws out energy—like adding
earth to a smoldering fire. It
effectively disengages us from
the source of intensity or agitation.

IRRITATED

Irritability occurs when we encounter something that disrupts our homeostasis. It can stem from not getting needs met, being in pain, or simply from another's disregard of our wellbeing. Sometimes, its causes are out of our control, which can lead to lashing out or being on the verge of full-blown anger.

Larimar

Larimar sets in motion the feelings of patience and peace. It acts as a bridge to shift from being irritated to feeling calm. This stone's visual appeal is a great reminder of the energy it provides; the cleansing power of a tranquil sea. Larimar cultivates you to build the skills necessary to manage stress and anxiety.
Try this: Sound and Stone Practice

Amazonite

Amazonite allows you to ease up the reigns of control with a gentle reassurance. It assists you to communicate without being clouded by irritation. This stone's compassionate nature validates feelings and helps you develop clear, concise conversations moving forward.
Try this: Touchstone Practice

Danburite

Danburite acts as a great emotional mediator. It links the higher self to the emotional body, cutting through irritation by connecting to the clear cause or underlying issue. It opens communication to receive guidance from the higher self. Danburite fosters the practice of consulting your inner wise one for insight and solutions.
Try this: Journaling Exercise

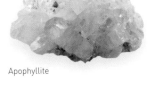
Apophyllite

Apophyllite

Apophyllite is an acute and gracious teacher. If we are feeling irritable, on edge, or on the verge of spinning out of control, this stone's frequency matches the intensity of the experience. This stone is like an energetic whirlpool stirring strongly in order to guide you back into the current of a coherent mental and emotional state.
Try this: Sound and Stone Practice

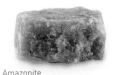
Amazonite

Powerful Stone Combinations	Danburite + Apophyllite
	Larimar + Pink Halite
	Amazonite + Apophyllite

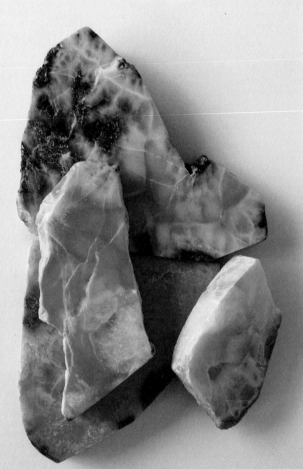

MORE
CRYSTALS
TO TRY

Pink Halite

Hemimorphite

Lithium Quartz

Larimar's tranquil
energy is emanated
in its beautiful
blue colors and
cool surface. It
navigates pathways
into patience to find
peace in prickly
situations.

NEEDY

Neediness exposes the tendency to look outside of ourselves for attention, comfort, and connection. While these needs are relevant and vital to the human condition, we can develop an unhealthy codependency, and if they are not being met properly, we may be left with a feeling of anxiety, insecurity, or abandonment.

Blue Apatite

Blue Apatite's energy is like a trusted friend or confidant. When you resonate with this stone, it lends support and helps you to discern what is behind neediness and how to proactively get your needs met.
Try this: Journaling Exercise

Sodalite

Sodalite reminds you to take care of your own needs first, so you may be helpful to others. It teaches you to manage inner resources well so you can show up to situations and relationships in life in a state of overflow rather than depletion. This stone helps to wash away insecurities or fears so you can implement healthy self-care.
Try this: Touchstone Practice

Obsidian

Obsidian helps you to take the time to understand and process your needs. It provides a protective space to settle into the depth of needy behaviors without fear of them. The asset of this stone's energy mirrors its creation from lava to natural glass. Obsidian teaches you how to shapeshift, and stand independently and strong. In return, you gain a new respect and reverence for your needs.
Try this: Sound and Stone Practice

Sunstone

Sunstone shines radiant light on the places in the body, mind, and soul that need attention. It activates personal power and works to remove scarcity thinking into abundance consciousness. In regards to relationships, Sunstone teaches you to practice making direct requests and allows the other party to meet you where they are willing and able.
Try this: Core Meditation Practice

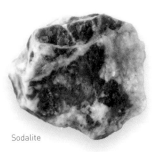

Sodalite

Powerful Stone Combinations

Obsidian + Blue Apatite
Obsidian + Sodalite
Obsidian + Sunstone

MORE
CRYSTALS
TO TRY

Hematite

Morganite

Dravite

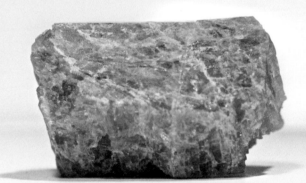

Blue Apatite
stimulates the
mind, allowing
us to identify and
communicate what
we are emotionally
longing for within
ourselves.

POSSESSIVE

Possessiveness comes from a desire to have control over something or someone. As it demands attention and consumes energy, possessiveness can cling so tightly, stifling the very thing we may be attempting to keep. It dominates our emotional landscape in an attempt to force destiny.

Tiger's Eye

Tiger's Eye teaches you how to find emotional balance. It centers the emotional body into equilibrium so you have the power to connect with your inner truth. It particularly helps compose thoughts and feelings around emotions that carry a strong charge or attachment.
Try this: Movement Meditation

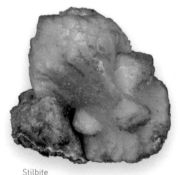

Stilbite

Blue Kyanite

Blue Kyanite quickly severs attachments to unwanted behaviors that isolate or hoard attention and energy. It recalibrates your whole being like a spark of light riding up and down the spine, as it sweeps away dense areas in the body where emotions have become trapped. Kyanite is a true gift-giver, teaching total freedom in abandoning the notion of control over resources, people, and possessions.
Try this: Core Meditation Practice

Stilbite

Stilbite deeply softens the body and mind, delivering mental clarity to shed light on what you are fiercely clinging onto in life. Its vibration allows you to open up to the opportunities of understanding and tolerance. At the same time, this stone encourages you to go deeper into knowing yourself without judgment.
Try this: Touchstone Practice

Sugilite

Sugilite severs old patterns of attachment that can constrict you into emotional pain. It helps remodel the areas of the body that may have been wounded by objectification. Sugilite teaches self-care, appreciating the little things in life, and valuing what is beyond the surface.
Try this: Conscious Crystal Dreaming

Powerful Stone Combinations	Blue Kyanite + Sugilite
	Stilbite + Tiger's Eye
	Stilbite + Sugilite

MORE
CRYSTALS
TO TRY

Ocean Jasper

Opal

Quartz

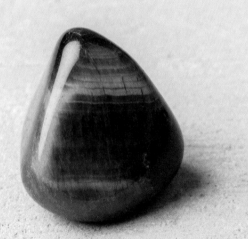

Tiger's Eye's
penetrating golden
vibrance carries
insight to aid us
in redirecting and
asserting our energy
to realign with our
genuine true nature.

FRUSTRATED

Frustration arises when an overwhelming feeling meets an internal stagnation. It is as if there is power inside without motion toward the goal. Once we can identify the underlying problem, see the goal, and channel that frustration into action; it becomes tinder upon the fire that moves us onward.

MORE
CRYSTALS
TO TRY

Serpentine

Snowflake
Obsidian (no
crystal structure)

Petrified Wood

Aquamarine

Aquamarine has a lightly flowing energy to call upon when you need to stop and calm down. A tool of contemplation and reflection, it can help you gain an outside perspective as the observer. This stone facilitates good communication with whatever healthy boundary you are trying to create.
Try this: Core Meditation Practice

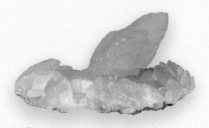

Dog Tooth Calcite

Dog Tooth Calcite

The energy of Dog Tooth Calcite allows frustrations to melt into the earth. Like rings of a tree, this stone echoes lessons of continual growth. It releases new information into awareness, allowing a shift in perspective. Like a hawk sitting in the highest of branches, this stone delivers insight into the areas that may need change for maximum growth.
Try this: Sound and Stone Practice

Amethyst

Amethyst clears the mind of the story that is creating chaos, acting as an elevator between the heart and mind and strengthening emotional intelligence. Its frequency moves you from rigidity and into the purification of the heart, helping you to overcome frustration by facilitating positive, gentle forward movement.
Try this: Touchstone Practice

Powerful Stone Combinations

Aquamarine + Amethyst
Serpentine + Amethyst
Serpentine + Dog Tooth Calcite

RESENTFUL

MORE
CRYSTALS
TO TRY

Pink Calcite

Amber (no
crystal structure)

Seraphinite

Resentment stems from the feeling that something is unjust or from not feeling fully appreciated. It can taint our ability to experience true happiness. Past pains and bitterness may keep bringing us back to the old place of wounds, rather than appreciating the present as an opportunity to create new and positive experiences.

Ruby
Resentment can be like knots in a string, and Ruby has an uncoiling effect, so energy can flow unobstructed. It ignites life force and unlocks areas in the body that are stagnant, promoting the free flow of energy in the body. This stone flushes out and cleanses, leaving you feeling better than before.
Try this: Movement Meditation

Green Tourmaline
Green Tourmaline emanates love. When you are feeling grievances hanging over you, this stone summons you to go deep into your heart. It can help you see where you have been blinded by the feelings of resentment. This stone restores your totality and helps you recognize how you are a valuable asset to family or community.
Try this: Core Meditation Practice

Lepidolite
Lepidolite enables you to choose to leave resentment behind. This proactive stone can be carried into difficult situations to avoid developing feelings of resentment. It helps you get to the heart of a situation without bringing the baggage that got you there. It offers acceptance and opens the throat to clear communication, allowing love to speak.
Try this: Touchstone Practice

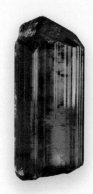

Green Tourmaline

Powerful Stone Combinations | Ruby + Pink Calcite
Green Tourmaline + Lepidolite

CHAPTER 5

CRYSTALS FOR INTUITIVE EMOTIONS

This chapter identifies emotions associated with the more intuitive aspects of one's self. It describes 12 different emotional states, some of which may be difficult to get in touch with—try one of the suggested exercises to help you engage with your emotion through a stone.

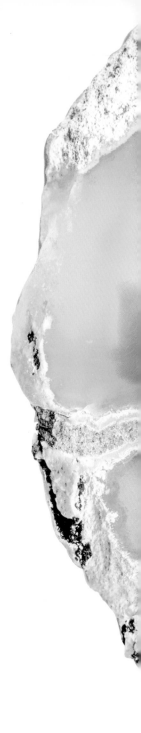

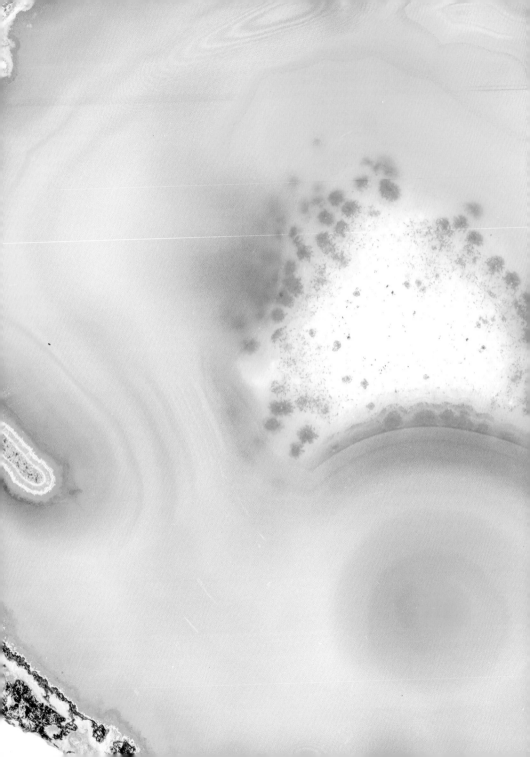

LOVING

Love is the strongest, most powerful, universal emotion humans possess. Unconditional love is wholesome, expansive, and knows no limitation. There are various manifestations of love and each of them share the simple aspect of connection. Love is a feeling that awakens the body energetically and is built upon trust.

Rose Quartz

Rose Quartz is a cardinal love crystal. When you are feeling disconnected from or not open to receiving love, this stone has the power to initiate a spark of light to activate and open the heart. Its tenacious energy can immediately be detected as it awakens the body to relax and surrender into the joy of unconditional love.
Try this: Sound and Stone Practice

Green Calcite

The calmness of Green Calcite encapsulates the exceptional healing intelligence that is inherently programmed into the Earth and its beings. This stone can help you explore your life purpose as it enhances the ability to practice deep

listening. Its frequency is a constant reminder to come back to a state of love.
Try this: Core Meditation Practice

Kunzite

Kunzite's pulsing energy opens the valves to the heart, creating subtle shifts to release any obstructions and let love flow in. This stone brings you back to fully cherishing the sacred privilege of life. It shifts perspective to lock you deep into remembering what you have to share with the world, no matter how big or small it may be.
Try this: Conscious Crystal Dreaming

Rubellite Tourmaline

Rubellite's energy communicates the message to the brain to fully trust your heart. This stone has the power to temporarily shrink down a problem or circumstance and fiercely bathe it in its never-ending light. Over time, Rubellite trains you to lead with the heart, then with the mind to stay centered and balanced. It brings solace to spaces that are still tender from old wounds of mistrust.
Try this: Touchstone Practice

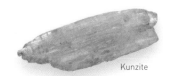

Kunzite

Powerful Stone Combinations	Pink Calcite + Rubellite
	Green Calcite + Pink Sapphire
	Rose Quartz + Kunzite

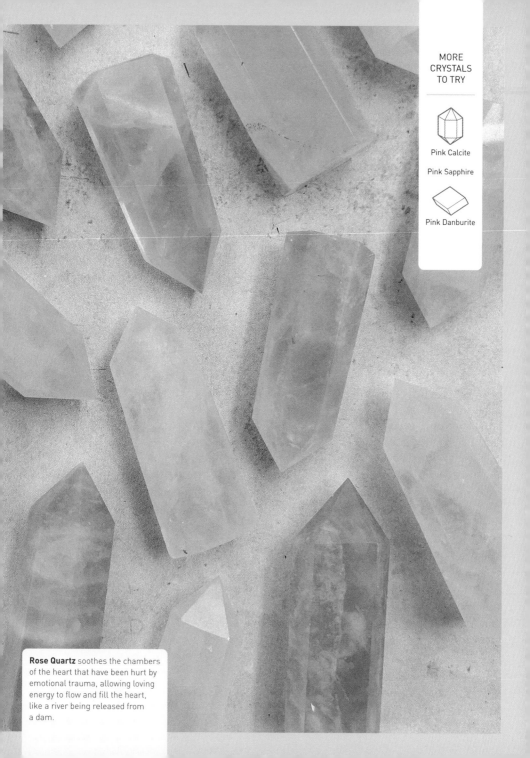

MORE
CRYSTALS
TO TRY

Pink Calcite

Pink Sapphire

Pink Danburite

Rose Quartz soothes the chambers of the heart that have been hurt by emotional trauma, allowing loving energy to flow and fill the heart, like a river being released from a dam.

EMPATHETIC

Empathy allows us to have an understanding of what another person is experiencing. Empathetic people are sensitive and aware of energies emanated by people or the environment around them. However, sometimes the energy can be felt acutely in the body and we may absorb too much of another person's pain or trauma.

Hemimorphite

Hemimorphite is a great ally for an overly empathetic person. It resonates with feminine strength and the cycles of the moon, teaching you to hone into the power of cyclical purification. This stone helps you learn techniques to prevent taking on other people's emotions or pain. It maintains your resilience through this practice of regeneration.
Try this: Touchstone Practice

Chrysanthemum Stone

Chrysanthemum Stone is a crystal of duality, bridging the two sides to every story. If you feel resistant to empathizing with a person or situation, it allows you to see a different perspective. This stone connects you to deep heart knowing, counterbalancing the mind from perpetuating a potentially biased perspective.
Try this: Sound and Stone Practice

Spinel

Spinel is a strong purifier, removing the dense areas in the emotional body caused by negative thinking. When resonating with this stone, you can find a deeper connection to self-compassion. It helps sift through and identify emotions, so you can pick which energy to engage in. Spinel also helps with practicing non-attachment.
Try this: Core Meditation Practice

Pink Halite

Pink Halite possesses a detoxifying purification for the mental and emotional body. It gently draws things to the surface to be cleansed away. This stone's youthful nature diverts rigid thinking by encouraging you to focus on shared commonalities in the human experience, rather than what separates individuals.
Try this: Touchstone Practice

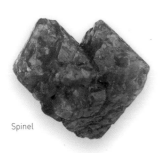

Spinel

Powerful Stone Combinations

Pink Halite + Cobalto Calcite
Chrysanthemum Stone + Hemimorphite
Lemurian Seed Crystal + Spinel

Hemimorphite opens us up to the latent power within receptivity and gives us the ability to connect with a deeper level of empathy for ourselves.

MORE
CRYSTALS
TO TRY

Rhodonite

Cobalto Calcite

Lemurian
Seed Crystal

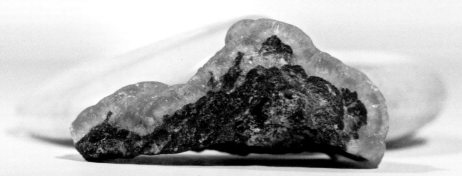

AT PEACE

Inner peace is something that lives, breathes, and grows within practices that nourish the mind, body, and spirit. Cultivation of inner peace carries us during tumultuous times and is a wave we make the choice to ride. We can choose to maintain emotional calmness in spite of tension or discord.

Selenite

The energy of Selenite looks after wellbeing. It resonates with realms of the mind, intuition, and spirit, and offers a protective cocoon of communication, helping to provide a clear channel to intuition or when connecting with spirit guides. This stone's high vibration has the ability to clear heavy energy and is a wonderful companion to lift you up when you are feeling down.
Try this: Movement Meditation

Rose Quartz

Rose Quartz is a great teacher when your inner peace is feeling vulnerable to disruption from outside influences. This stone energetically works to effectively supply the emotional body with a sense of deep serenity. Its fast-acting frequency helps you easily shift from sensitivity into certainty.
Try this: Touchstone Practice

Dioptase

Dioptase cuts through self-imposed limitations to access the parts of the self that are numb. This stone makes an opening where energy can become readily available and increases the quality

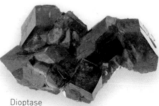
Dioptase

of that energy. It entrains your emotional being with greater feelings of fulfillment. Dioptase guides you to find the opportunities to function in a healthier way and act gradually to make improvements.
Try this: Core Meditation Practice

Emerald

Emerald vibrates with the theme of deep perseverance. It sits in the core of your being to show where growth is needed and helps to bring peace to the emotional body by developing a greater connection with Earth's frequencies.
Try this: Journaling Exercise

Powerful Stone Combinations	Rose Quartz + Emerald
	Selenite + Hiddenite
	Dioptase + Larimar

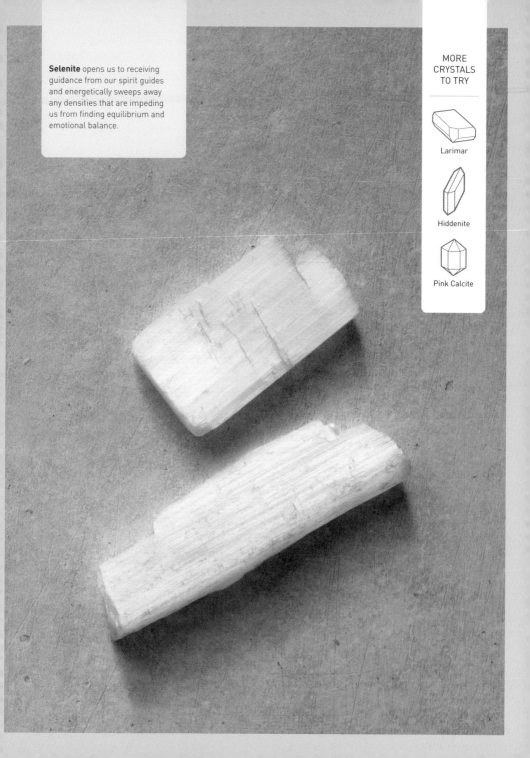

Selenite opens us to receiving guidance from our spirit guides and energetically sweeps away any densities that are impeding us from finding equilibrium and emotional balance.

MORE CRYSTALS TO TRY

Larimar

Hiddenite

Pink Calcite

JOYFUL

When we pay attention, there is a lot to celebrate within the simplicities of life. Witnessing a small act of kindness, sharing laughter with a loved one, or paying a bill on time, are various forms of joy. Focusing on the positive aspects of life promotes more experiences of receiving joyful pleasure.

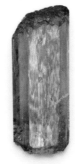

Hiddenite

Lepidolite

When feeling blocked from happiness, Lepidolite whispers, "Keep going! The payoff is huge!" This stone is a charmer, with its great encouragement to keep moving forward even when you are encountering resistance or want to give up. It guides you to check in on inner energy reserves and collaboratively works to help fill your inner well to promote emotional wellbeing.
Try this: Sound and Stone Practice

Hiddenite

Hiddenite builds self-confidence and conjures fool-like innocence to express itself. This stone will remind you to not take life too seriously and to lighten up through spontaneous play. It is a stone of adventure as it inspires you to connect to the joy found in the journey not the outcome.
Try this: Touchstone Practice

Gold

As a precious metal, the frequency of gold transports you to embody a liveliness and indulgence to live life fully. It is synonymous with abundance and teaches you how to resonate with its generous message. The synergy of gold with crystals or minerals has a lavishing effect on the physical and emotional body and delights all who carry it.
Try this: Core Meditation Practice

Chrysanthemum Stone

Chrysanthemum Stone is a reminder of the simple joys of life. You can find beauty between the cracks of concrete on a city street or life purpose in surviving a painful situation. This stone is a catalyst to help you find a small sliver of light even in the darkest places.
Try this: Movement Meditation

Powerful Stone Combinations	Hiddenite + Gold
	Lepidolite + Chrysanthemum Stone
	Lepidolite + Gold

Lepidolite gives the mind an extra push to flash forward into the heart of joy. Its energetic effect acts like a sneak preview of immediate satisfaction and happiness.

MORE
CRYSTALS
TO TRY

Chalcedony

Heliodor

Citrine

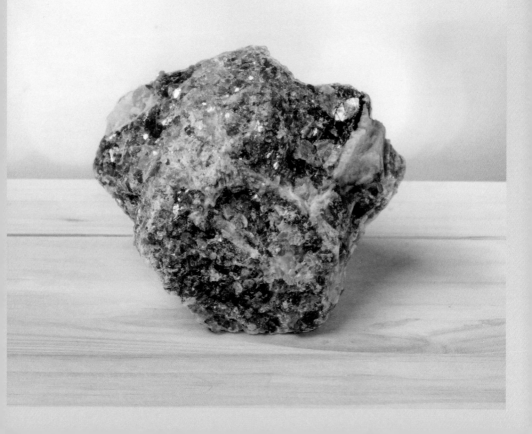

BLISSFUL

Bliss is the feeling of being on top of the world, giving us the experience of pure elation. It is as if our awareness has been fine-tuned and the synchronicities in life are magnified. Bliss is seeing the beauty in everything, living our best life and celebrating it.

Moonstone

Moonstone is a very mystical and powerful crystal that drives you deeper down the spiral of life learning. It teaches the duality between light and dark, and aids in understanding how these polarities provide a wholesome life experience. This stone keeps you on the path of personal growth and reinvention, illuminating higher perspectives and connecting you to greater life purpose.
Try this: Conscious Crystal Dreaming

Green Jade

Green Jade resonates with prosperity and good luck. It brings you deep into the heart center and increases the heart's capacity to receive love, bliss, and joy. This stone reveals the true nature of abundance without attachment to material things.
Try this: Sound and Stone Practice

Ocean Jasper

Ocean Jasper casts a soothing effect on the mind, body, and spirit when they are filled with anger, resentment, or pain. Its frequency exudes a cavernous serenity to connect you to deep ease. This stone directs attention to your grounding cord to send dense energies into the Earth to be restored. Ocean Jasper opens the doors to let joy overflow in your life again.
Try this: Touchstone Practice

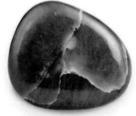

Green Jade

Powerful Stone Combinations	Turquoise + Jade Blue Apatite + Moonstone

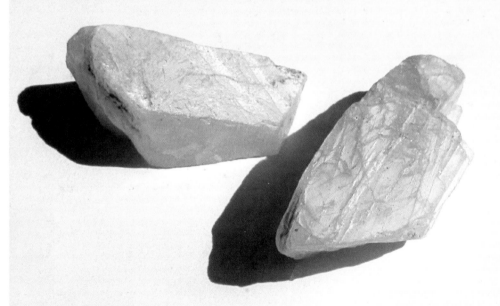

MORE
CRYSTALS
TO TRY

Sugilite

Blue Apatite

Turquoise

Moonstone uplifts us with
the energy of joy and invites
synchronicity into everyday
life. It affirms our intuition and
asserts us to celebrate the
interconnectedness of life.

COMPASSIONATE

Being compassionate allows us to view things through another person's perspective and gives us an undeniable drive to initiate action to help. Our feelings of compassion serve as an advocate to help release the burden of another's suffering.

Rhodochrosite

Rhodochrosite lifts the fog, giving insight to explore inner areas that lack compassion for the self and others. This stone offers a new perspective and gives you the courage to take action and practice forgiveness. It heeds you to stay aware and keep coming back to love and acceptance of the self and others.
Try this: Movement Meditation

Grossular Garnet

Grossular Garnet acts as a mentor or counselor to guide you to make the necessary changes and actions to live a compassionate life. It steers you in the right direction to find and solve injustices. This stone is a great asset for any collaboration as it strengthens the bonds that tether humanity together.
Try this: Conscious Crystal Dreaming

Seraphinite

Seraphinite takes you on a pilgrimage into the depths of the soul to look at all aspects of your life with loving kindness. This stone helps call on inner wisdom to be guided by the forces of love and compassion. It activates the notion that no one is alone and can request support from seen and unseen sources.
Try this: Touchstone Practice

Peridot

Peridot radiates hope. When the heart is closed due to past trauma, or habitual self-hatred, it alleviates pain. Its light green color creates a waterfall of compassion in the heart, allowing the old patterns to flow away with the current. It puts the inner bully to bed, and reprograms the emotional body with new references to build upon.
Try this: Journaling Exercise

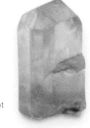

Peridot

Powerful Stone Combinations	Peridot + Seraphinite
	Rhodochrosite + Grossular Garnet

MORE
CRYSTALS
TO TRY

Honey Calcite

Pink Tourmaline

Serpentine

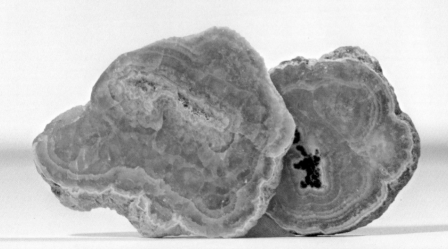

Rhodochrosite delivers a
warmhearted crystalline energy to
generously nurture the emotional
body, especially for those who tend
to be overly harsh or critical of
themselves or others.

DISAPPOINTED

Disappointment elicits a feeling of unhappiness between our hopes and intentions and what actually materializes into reality. We are often left with a bitter taste of defeat or failure and the feeling of disappointment can be a setback to our resilience. We are asked to reexamine the relationship of expectations.

Red Coral

Red Coral pushes you to dive deep beyond the surface of your existence. It illuminates behaviors in which you are looking outside of yourself for happiness or fixated on a thing that is perceived to bring happiness. Instead, this stone explicitly teaches you how to focus on the feelings of what is desired, to move with confidence and heart-knowing toward that feeling.

Try this: Movement Meditation

Gold Sheen Obsidian

Gold Sheen Obsidian can mend the emotional frayed edges caused by disappointment. This stone's energy provides a feeling of safety and protection. It offers the perspective to see possible ways around obstacles that derailed a path you may have felt attached to. It teaches you to abandon conditions you may have projected onto your desires that may be limiting to overall success.

Try this: Touchstone Practice

Imperial Topaz

Imperial Topaz ignites the fire of personal will when the wind has blown out your candle. The fire energy present in this stone acts as a spotlight, revealing the areas that are vulnerable and need to be rebuilt and tended to. When you are struggling to meet your needs or goals, this stone provides the motivation to proceed and pursue what you are trying to achieve.

Try this: Core Meditation Practice

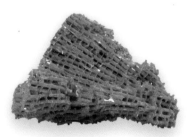

Red Coral

Powerful Stone Combinations	Gold Sheen Obsidian + Red Coral
	Lapis Lazuli + Amber
	Dravite + Golden Topaz

MORE
CRYSTALS
TO TRY

Amber
(no crystal
structure)

Dravite

Lapis Lazuli
(no crystal
structure)

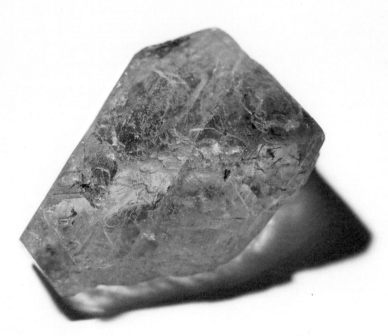

Imperial Topaz is a stone of cheer
and delight, shining its warm light
to fill our happiness cup that may
feel on the verge of being empty.

HOPELESS

Hopelessness relies on habitual negative thought patterns that reinforce, promote, or perhaps even prove that circumstances or situations will not change. Hopelessness isolates and disconnects us from the source of creation. When we feel hopeless, we feel lost in the world and we do not know where to fit into society or community.

Black Kyanite

Black Kyanite alleviates the burdens you carry. This stone quickly initiates a transference of energy, ushering out the old and welcoming in the new. It emanates the power of truth and certainty, catapulting you across new planes of existence. When feeling hopeless, Black Kyanite breaks you free of negative thought patterns, enhancing protection so healthy thinking becomes much clearer.
Try this: Movement Meditation

Moonstone

Moonstone invites you to connect and reflect on life's purpose. It has the ability to shine light within the areas that have long been neglected.

This stone enables you to work with the shadow self without fear. It attracts more beauty and joy to radiate into your life, fueling the power to show up for yourself wholly.
Try this: Core Meditation Practice

Green Fluorite

Green Fluorite takes the edge off over-thinking or analyzing, giving you permission to be playful and creative. It aids you to complete goals, allowing the feelings of accomplishment to grow. When you are feeling hopeless and inadequate, Green Fluorite is a reminder that sometimes the most profound shifts can occur during total chaos.
Try this: Conscious Crystal Dreaming

Galena

Galena is a powerhouse of wisdom and is excellent at pulling us out of the funk of life. This stone has the ability to jolt you into the next part of the healing journey to move forward again. Galena helps hone and repair the parts of the emotional body that have been fragmented due to emotional trauma. It reminds you that help is readily obtainable.
Try this: Sound and Stone Practice

Powerful Stone Combinations | Moonstone + Hematite
Galena + Rose Quartz

MORE
CRYSTALS
TO TRY

Hematite

Petrified Wood

Rose Quartz

Black Kyanite lurches us out of dark places in the mind to orbit us into a new reality of possibility or circumstance.

MOURNFUL

Mourning is the emotional process we experience and express to release and heal from loss of any kind. We may mourn the loss of a loved one, a trauma, or even the loss of an identity, or a part of our life that is no longer present.

Aquamarine

Aquamarine is an emotionally charged stone that carries the energy of the ocean or moving body of water. This stone allows you the space to be alone and mourn whatever the loss is at the time. It brings comfort in the same way a beautiful song does to a broken heart. Aquamarine opens you up to being more receptive to receiving help from others.
Try this: Touchstone Practice

Rose Quartz

The soothing energy of Rose Quartz can help you feel safe enough to release what is laying heavy on your heart. This stone is a wonderful companion in times of deep loss and allows you to honor and surrender to what you cannot control. It opens up areas in the emotional body that are withholding the true expression of grief without being consumed by it.
Try this: Sound and Stone Practice

Emerald

Emerald has the energy of new birth to assist you in moving out of feelings of mourning or grief. It nurtures you back to life, inspiring purpose and a connectedness to all things. This crystal relates to the heart of the matter at hand, aiding you with the ability to return to love once again.
Try this: Core Meditation Practice

Pink Halite

Pink Halite is like having the cleansing ocean in your fingertips. It encourages you to lay the sorrow weighing on the heart in the landscape of the stone. Its vibration soothingly washes over the emotional body like words written in the sand as waves lap over it, leaving you feeling lighter and more buoyant, yet supported.
Try this: Touchstone Practice

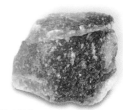

Pink Halite

Powerful Stone Combinations	Rose Quartz + Black Tourmaline
	Gold + Emerald
	Pink Halite + Aquamarine

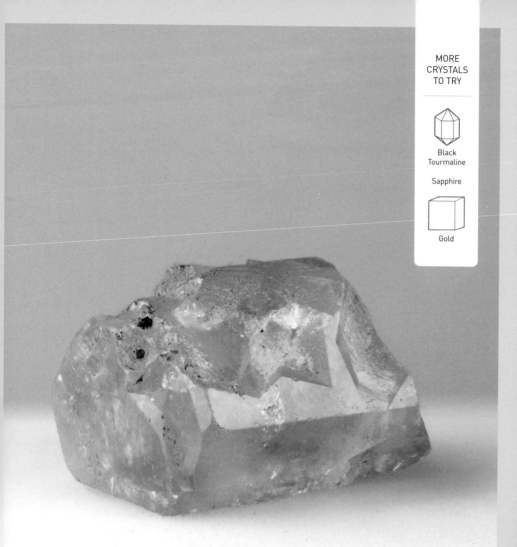

MORE
CRYSTALS
TO TRY

Black
Tourmaline

Sapphire

Gold

Aquamarine conjures the ability to
let go and communicates a healthy
sense of relief found in the power
of release.

SHAMEFUL

Shame is a deflating emotion that exposes a failure to meet up to some standard set in society and is fueled by feelings of unworthiness or never being good enough. The self-blame of shame is taxing on the spirit and can leave us vulnerable to a feeling of wanting to shrink away or disappear entirely.

Pyrite

Pyrite meets you where you are on your healing journey. It helps you reflect and examine the cracks living within your foundation. If shame is living in those spaces, Pyrite aids in strength and courage to face that shame with love from the core of your being. Pyrite renews and awakens you to your potential, aids your self-awareness, and helps you to see a new path in life.
Try this: Conscious Crystal Dreaming

Stibnite

Stibnite is the fast track to the truth. It has the unique ability to obliterate the nonsense and falseness to reveal things as they truly are. This stone gives you the courage to admit any perceived shortcomings or fears of inadequacy without the emotional attachment to them.
Try this: Touchstone Practice

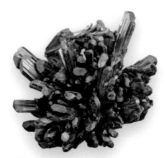

Stibnite

Mahogany Obsidian

Mahogany Obsidian teaches you to bask in exploration of the self and recognize the beauty that lies within. It can cut through shame like a sword to reveal a deeper understanding of its root cause. This stone severs the loop of negative thought patterns and invites you to wholeheartedly believe in yourself and focus on the value you bring.
Try this: Core Meditation Practice

Powerful Stone Combinations	Stibnite + Lepidolite Azurite + Mahogany Obsidian + Lemurian Jade

Azurite

Lemurian Jade

Lepidolite

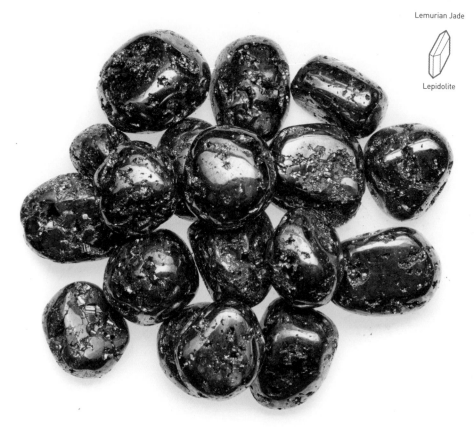

Pyrite acts as a mirror to help us
examine our own personal stigmas
and transform these experiences
into strength to fortify the totality of
our emotional wellbeing.

DISCOURAGED

Discouragement halts progress—it is like the wind being taken out of our sails. The experience is quite the dampener on the spirit and when we fall short of what we anticipated we are left feeling uncertain. Discouragement elicits self-doubt to creep in and causes us to question whether we were on the right path to begin with.

Wulfenite

Wulfenite helps shield you from outside influences that affect your confidence. When you are feeling down or out, this stone will lend the self-assurance you need to take action and climb up the ladder of life again. Wulfenite helps you step out of discouragement and into a renewed passion for life.
Try this: Core Meditation Practice

Tiger's Eye

Tiger's Eye carries a stimulating energy like a coach who gets the team pumped before a game. Its energy encapsulates the animalistic and determined nature of a tiger, giving you the courage to go after what you desire. This stone brings you home to the strength of your will, and your own personal power and inner truth.
Try this: Movement Meditation Practice

Faden Quartz

Faden Quartz mends the emotional aspects of yourself that have been shattered due to disappointment. This stone stimulates you to grow in new directions following discouragement, and teaches you perseverance and determination.
Try this: Conscious Crystal Dreaming

Selenite

Selenite has the power of a forceful wind to clear the channels of the mind. It sweeps away discouraging thoughts to put an end to doubt or anxiety. This stone's wild nature brings fresh optimistic feelings, promising a sense of renewed ambition. Working with this crystal invokes a connectedness to something greater.
Try this: Sound and Stone Practice

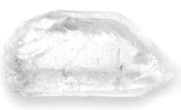

Selenite

Powerful Stone Combinations	Tiger's Eye + Selenite Wulfenite + Faden Quartz

MORE
CRYSTALS
TO TRY

Onyx

Carnelian

Amazonite

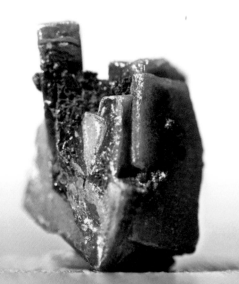

Wulfenite burns away stagnation
and jumpstarts the will center
with renewed determination and
persistence to pursue our efforts
and undertakings.

SORROWFUL

Sorrow can feel like being trapped in a trench of sadness, withdrawn from the joys of life. It may stem from the loss of someone or be rooted in a feeling of being on the outside. Sorrow can make us feel perpetually stuck in a rut and lead to depression.

Amber

Amber moves energy like sap, slowly and steadily, giving you the ability to fully feel the emotion in order to let go and lay it down. This stone can also trap unwanted feelings in its resin, making space for clarity and truth. Amber has the ability to dispel depression and help you return to being with others and finding a sense of purpose.
Try this: Touchstone Practice

Celestine

Celestine lovingly plugs you into a boundless portal of spiritual healing. It invigorates the soul and gently sparks life into the totality of your being. Celestine teaches you how to sit with the uncomfortable feelings of sorrow and pain as an observer. It empowers you to walk through the storms of life and come out the other side with greater perspective and self-knowing.
Try this: Core Meditation Practice

Shiva Lingam

Shiva Lingam's ancient energy connects to the web of light and support available through your lineage. Resonating with this stone reinforces the feelings of not being alone in sorrow. It encourages you

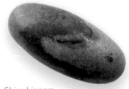

Shiva Lingam

to call on and lean into that energetic support.
Try this: Movement Meditation

Chrysocolla

Chrysocolla is a crystal that helps you connect to equanimity. It fosters peaceful exploration of your inner landscape, allowing personal suffering to be fully processed and released. At the same time, this stone becomes a pipeline to reestablishing a new relationship with yourself that is free from any distress of the past.
Try this: Journaling Exercise

Powerful Stone Combinations	Shiva Lingam + Rhodonite Celestine + Chrysocolla Amber + Bloodstone

Desert Rose

Rhodonite

Bloodstone

Amber's light and non-abrasive
nature provides a gentle frequency
to the emotional body. Its rich,
radiant color has the power to
brighten up our being even in the
difficulties of our darkest days.

CHAPTER 6

CRYSTALS FOR
MENTAL CLARITY

This chapter identifies emotions associated
with the more interior aspects of one's mind.
It describes 12 different emotional states, and
a suggested practical ritual to enrich your
life and achieve insight and self-knowledge.

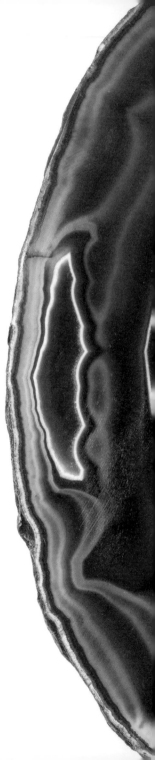

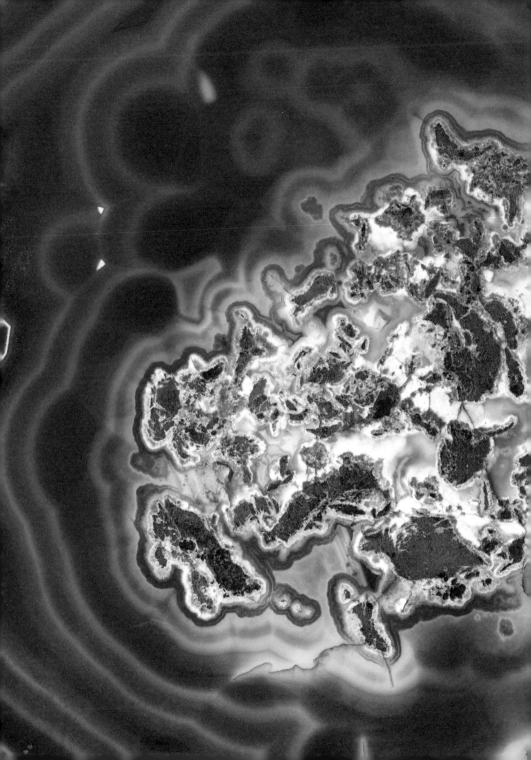

ENLIGHTENED

The mental state of enlightenment promises a deeper purpose in life. It lives intimately in the present moment to help us overcome adversity, transcend the ego, and find peace through the polarizing beauty, darkness, pain, or suffering that accompanies life. Enlightenment peels away labels to reveal the raw essence of the divine self and soul.

Spirit Quartz

Spirit Quartz is a stone of refuge that opens you up to receptivity and growth. It helps you understand the power of the present moment, cutting through limitations of the mind and connecting you to the vast networks of consciousness available beyond the self. It offers comfort and a deeper comprehension of the power of love and compassion.
Try this: Sound and Stone Practice

Cinnabar

Cinnabar is a messenger between dimensional realities, linking you to the alchemical process of transformation. It pushes out limiting patterns, attuning you to higher states of awareness. Cinnabar can open pathways to abundance acting as leverage into maintaining emotional prosperity and wealth of knowledge.
Try this: Core Meditation Practice

Fulgurite

Fulgurite carries the energy of enlightenment. It will burst through any glass ceiling and enchant you to embark on an expedition into the soul and has the power to conjure a storm to purify the emotional body. Its unique hollow structure carries intentions into the winds with lightning speed to help manifest hopes and dreams.
Try this: Touchstone Practice

Moldavite

Moldavite delivers new ways of thinking and acting, expanding the mind without set limits or boundaries. Its intense frequency breaks apart outdated belief systems, transporting you into a deeper understanding of life and beyond.
Try this: Core Meditation Practice

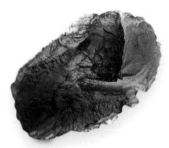

Moldavite

Powerful Stone Combinations	Moldavite + Fulgurite
	Spirit Quartz + Cinnabar
	Cinnabar + Fulgurite

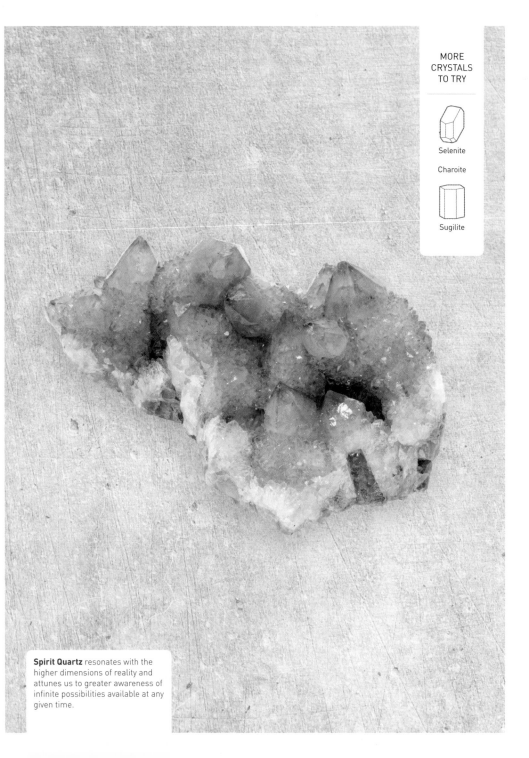

MORE
CRYSTALS
TO TRY

Selenite

Charoite

Sugilite

Spirit Quartz resonates with the
higher dimensions of reality and
attunes us to greater awareness of
infinite possibilities available at any
given time.

INSPIRED

Like the arrival of springtime when nature is actively budding with new life and fertility, the feeling of being inspired encapsulates a clean emotional slate. Inspiration frees us from past limitations and a plethora of potential lives within its growth, undoubtedly propelling us forward.

MORE
CRYSTALS
TO TRY

Quartz

Lemurian Seed
Crystal

Fluorite

Tibetan Black Quartz

Tibetan Black Quartz resonates with personal freedom and how to inspire freedom in your community and collective world. This stone showcases the myriad of sources you may draw on for inspiration. It also removes stagnation through its double termination structure, moving energy in different directions.
Try this: Journaling Exercise

Elestial Quartz

Elestial Quartz has the power to directly channel high-frequency energies. This stone connects the bands of the past, present, and future and even though it is incredibly grounding, it encourages

you to get out there and be proactive. It draws in positive energy and pushes out unwanted energy, creating a protective cocoon of space in which you can feel inspired.
Try this: Conscious Crystal Dreaming

Picture Jasper

Picture Jasper is an entryway to inspiration. It tells a vivid story within its unique visual landscapes and is wonderful for meditation and visualization. It evokes imagination and creativity to flow down through the lower energy centers, propelling you to stay self-motivated. This stone is incredibly grounding and at the same time rousing

for mental stimulation and connecting with your intuition.
Try this: Touchstone Practice

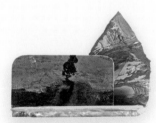

Picture jasper

Powerful Stone Combinations

Elestial Quartz + Quartz
Picture Jasper + Tibetan Black Quartz

LIBERATED

Emotional liberation reclaims the happiness that all human beings deserve to experience. It comes from a place of understanding other people's feelings without sacrificing our own emotional needs and wellbeing. The experience of emotional liberation allows us to explore the world with confidence and compassion in our own unique way.

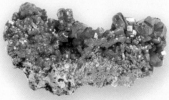

Vanadinite

Andalusite

Andalusite connects you directly to the feeling of liberation and deliverance. "X" literally marks the spot on the visible surface of a cut Andalusite crystal. Each direction of the cross-section contains its own healing rite. This stone takes you on a journey through themes of the emotional body—from survival and thriving into passion and creation, to love and bliss, and intuition and insight.
Try this: Journaling Exercise

Vanadinite

Vanadinite ignites the areas of truth that are not yet open for you to look at or deal with. This stone respectfully offers salvation to move through difficult emotional blocks, or repressed memories. As a true catalyst of change, Vanadinite gives you the courage to move through uncomfortable release into liberty and independence.
Try this: Movement Meditation

Sugilite

Sugilite reawakens you to get back in the driver's seat of life and find its simple joys. If you are expelling too much energy managing other people's emotions, this stone redirects that attention into taking care of yourself. It also encourages mutual relationships to be built on understanding and honoring each other's feelings without trying to fix anything.
Try this: Conscious Crystal Dreaming

Selenite

Selenite brings a feeling of comfort like a trusted friend. Anything you share with it remains sacred. This stone connects you to ancestors and guides, providing a feeling of being held and loved. It clears emotional space for the new; dissolving fear, anger, and misunderstanding.
Try this: Movement Meditation

Powerful Stone Combinations

Vanadinite + Selenite
Sugilite + Andalusite

INTELLECTUAL

Intellect is not limited to academia and being "book-smart"—there are multiple ways it can be expressed. Intellectual people are often creative, able to problem-solve, think outside the box, communicate well, and express a high level of emotional intelligence.

Azurite

Azurite encourages a more receptive and open mind. When you are able to expand the mind, the intellectual areas of the brain soften, allowing more information to be processed. This stone opens the pineal gland, influencing the brain to rest, but also stimulates you to connect with the less dominant side of the brain.
Try this: Sound and Stone Practice

Black Tourmaline

Black Tourmaline acts as a sponge, absorbing energies in the body that are holding tension. When you are heavily engaged in intellectual activities and your brain starts to feel depleted, this stone will invigorate you with a renewed sense of energy to restore the hunger to learn and stay focused.
Try this: Journaling Exercise

Green Apatite

Green Apatite connects to the areas of the mind that feel fatigued due to overuse. It connects the mind to the heart, allowing the intellectual aspects to rest in its sanctuary. Green Apatite is a great assistant for big projects or tests. It centers the mind and sparks enthusiasm, so you may find completion not depletion in all that you do.
Try this: Conscious Crystal Dreaming

Labradorite

Labradorite connects you to curiosity and spontaneity. It is a mystical stone and, like an elevator, it can bring you to a new doorway of awareness. It reveals alternative ways of intellectual thinking or challenges you to choose another path than the one you already know. When actively working with Labradorite, it may increase the flow of synchronicity into life.
Try this: Core Meditation Practice

Powerful Stone Combinations

Black Tourmaline + Labradorite
Blue Tourmaline + Azurite
Blue Apatite + Labradorite

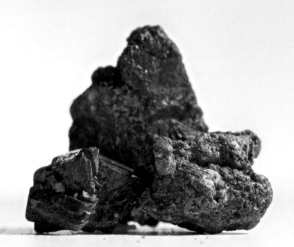

MORE
CRYSTALS
TO TRY

Apophyllite

Blue Apatite

Blue Tourmaline

Azurite gives access to the more obscure parts of consciousness and nurtures us to explore alternate ways of thinking and relating to the world around us.

SPIRITUAL

Being spiritual implies that there is something greater to life beyond what is witnessed at the surface. It is an interconnection to all parts of the whole, with an acute awareness of intuition and cultivating the ability to trust our instincts. Spiritual experiences rarely fit the conventional boxes society teaches and thereby move us into an experiential understanding of the world.

Amethyst

Amethyst is a helpful companion in looking at addictive behaviors and accepting responsibility for them. It peels back the layers behind the facade, giving you courage to look at the shadow self. Spiritually it is an essential stone in the healing process of addictive behaviors or substance abuse. It empowers you to practice self-forgiveness and shields you from any negative thought patterns.
Try this: Conscious Crystal Dreaming

Turquoise

Turquoise is a stone of awakening, love, connection, creativity, and depth. It has the ability to push you to a breaking point to create rapid change and growth. This stone shapeshifts you out of the old paradigm and onto a new platform of spiritual awakening. It can bring a level of discomfort if you are not ready to move forward into a spiritual quest.
Try this: Sound and Stone Practice

Lemurian Seed Crystal

Lemurian Seed Crystal carries the documentation of the Earth's records. It has the ability to transcend you beyond this reality. This stone brings human awareness into the different dimensional layers that make the fabric of this world. It awakens you to understand life is deep and filled with things you can't always experience with the tangible senses but can intuitively feel.
Try this: Movement Meditation

Green Apophyllite

Green Apophyllite's amplitude softens the breath and body to connect you to unseen forces. It invites the heart to open and listen to ancestral guidance. This stone clears the slate of fear and unhappiness in order to step fully onto a spiritual path. It sparks resilience and invites the imaginative self to step forward.
Try this: Conscious Crystal Dreaming

Powerful Stone Combinations	Turquoise + Lemurian Seed Crystal
	Red Coral + Turquoise
	Lapis Lazuli + Green Apophyllite

Amethyst is a dynamic pillar of support to explore the depths of spirituality and bridge the multidimensional realities of existence and our unique human experience.

MORE
CRYSTALS
TO TRY

Red Coral

Orange Kyanite

Lapis Lazuli
(no crystal
structure)

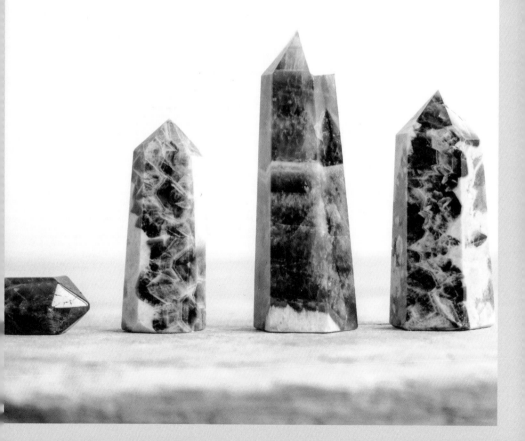

ATTRACTED

We feel uplifted when we are in the presence of, or communicating with, someone or something we feel attracted to. Attracting the things we want reflects where we are in our personal growth. Whether we are looking to attract a job, lover, friend, or home, we must first be clear in what feeling is desired and proceed with action to fulfill it.

Stibnite

Stibnite is a stone of great manifestation; it grounds the will center to bring to life what you are looking to attract. This stone matches the intensity of what you are ready and capable of achieving and you should be clear and direct when requesting help from it. Stibnite has the ability to reflect whatever is needed to walk a life filled with purpose.
Try this: Core Meditation Practice

Herkimer Diamond

Herkimer Diamond carries the message and understanding that you get back what you put in. Its energy bridges a clear path to attracting good fortune and success. Alternatively,

when you are on the wrong path, Herkimer Diamond holds the power to attract the proper action needed in order to keep you moving in the right direction.
Try this: Sound and Stone Practice

Magnetic Hematite

Magnetic Hematite grounds the high vibrations of the mind into the Earth, rooting your desires in the here and now. This stone draws things to the surface in order to release them and attract the new. It can also help to protect you from self-doubt.
Try this: Touchstone Practice

Faden Quartz

Faden Quartz attunes you to your truest vibrational state. It goes right to the root cause of an inability to attract dreams and prevent precious energy leakage. This stone will mend the area filled with uncertainty, allowing healing to take place. Faden Quartz loves to work in pairs. To dial up the intensity of its effects, try holding two stones together.
Try this: Sound and Stone Practice

Powerful Stone Combinations	Stibnite + Magnetic Hematite
	Herkimer Diamond + Stibnite

Stibnite's dynamic frequency both initiates and steeps into us over time. It magnetizes us when we are truly ready to take a big risk and fully leap into the next stage of our lives.

MORE
CRYSTALS
TO TRY

Obsidian
(no crystal
structure)

Amethyst

Spessartine
Garnet

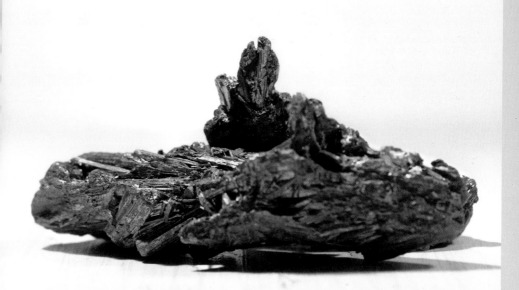

INSECURE

Insecurity emanates from a lack of self-confidence and may occur when we are harshly judged by ourselves or others, or from embedded emotional wounds of the past. When we are feeling insecure, it indicates a real need for self-love and care. We need to find a way to banish negative self-talk and self-doubt, and our dependency on others.

Carnelian

Carnelian gives you the self-belief to stand independently. When setting your mind on something, it feeds the fire to reassure you to take action to accomplish your goals. It torches self-sabotaging thoughts that might hinder you. *Try this: Touchstone Practice*

Larimar

Larimar washes away self-doubt in the sanctuary of love found deep within the recesses of the heart. If there is the tendency for energy to be solely directed toward one avenue or person, Larimar teaches you to open up to the myriad of other support systems available. This stone dissolves the notion of dependency on one area or person to get your needs met. *Try this: Sound and Stone Practice*

Sapphire

When feeling isolated, alone, or helpless, Sapphire's warrior-like energy gives you the tenacity to withstand turmoil or adversity. This stone helps expunge uncertainty to release fear or hesitation, and teaches you to honor yourself, to mute the inner critic, and to learn from your imperfections. *Try this: Movement Meditation*

Morganite

Morganite is a stone of the wounded healer, with the ability to enable great change. If you are not ready to release the wounds of the past, you will fester with insecurity. When you are willing to heal any limiting past traumas, this stone helps to bring compassion and love to fill that wound. It helps to foster a feeling of safety and assurance. *Try this: Core Meditation Practice*

Morganite

Powerful Stone Combinations	Larimar + Sapphire
	Morganite + Pink Tourmaline
	Emerald + Sapphire

MORE
CRYSTALS
TO TRY

Emerald

Aquamarine

Pink Tourmaline

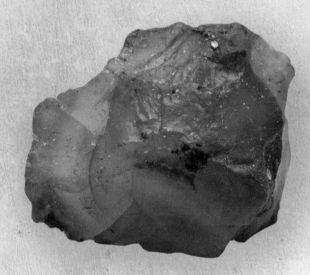

Carnelian's vibration is that of a
mighty oak tree, it offers stability
when we are feeling insecure
about our self-image, career,
or relationships.

GUILTY

Guilt is a huge vampire of our emotional wellbeing. It taxes the mind and spirit and can taint our self-concept. Although guilt is wired to the conscience to help discern wrongs of the past, it can crystallize and harden your ability to grow and move forward in life.

MORE
CRYSTALS
TO TRY

Obsidian
(no crystal
structure)

Garnet

Kunzite

Watermelon Tourmaline

Watermelon Tourmaline gracefully breaks the surface of an issue to gently chisel its way closer to the heart of the matter. It allows you a portal to climb through and the courage to discover what lies both above and beneath the surface. This stone generates warmth and invites the support needed to help you make amends.
Try this: Sound and Stone Practice

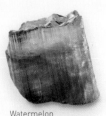

Watermelon
Tourmaline

Apache Tears

Apache Tears is a stone of absolution. It disrupts and helps release the tense grip of guilt on the emotional body and encourages you to give it over to the Earth as compost. When experiencing intense guilt, this stone lightens the emotional load you may carry and begins the process of reprogramming the psyche and practicing self-forgiveness for past mistakes.
Try this: Conscious Crystal Dreaming

Chrysocolla

Chrysocolla is a great friend to clear the murky waters of miscommunication. This stone allows you the space to objectively reflect on a situation to better process and understand it, without the stigma of guilt to cloud it. Chrysocolla gives you the competence to convey information or feelings, from the heart, not the head.
Try this: Core Meditation Practice

Andalusite

Andalusite teaches you to live, learn from experience, and let go. It is a stone of deep introspection. Andalusite also has the ability to cast a protective shell over the emotional body when you are feeling vulnerable to being manipulated or made to feel guilty about something.
Try this: Journaling Exercise

Powerful Stone Combinations

Andalusite + Apache Tears
Chrysocolla + Watermelon Tourmaline
Kunzite + Watermelon Tourmaline

CONFUSED

Feeling confused greatly hinders our ability to communicate and make decisions, and weakens our confidence. Confusion inhibits integration and severely degrades mental acuity. There is a disconnect from being present in your body when you are swept up in a whirlwind of emotions that upset self-awareness, and impact on your relationships and surroundings.

MORE
CRYSTALS
TO TRY

Mahogany
Obsidian
(no crystal
structure)

Blue Lace Agate

Blue Calcite

Clear Fluorite

Clear Fluorite is like the "undo" button on the emotional and mental body. Its frequency combs the mind to restore it back to its original nature. This stone also frees up mental capacity as it encourages you to release any excessive thoughts.
Try this: Core Meditation Practice

Danburite

Danburite is a stone to call on when you need to be refocused. When working in meditation, it gives you access to guidance, navigating you through the fog of confusion. This stone is a great tuner, facilitating you to clearly hear the messages or wisdom of your intuition.
Try this: Journaling Exercise

Amethyst

Amethyst connects you to a state of knowing. It stops the record of unproductive thoughts and helps you get "unstuck," providing a pathway to usable active energy. It removes brain fog to bring clarity and can be transformational for deep brain healing and improved mental functioning.
Try this: Conscious Crystal Dreaming

Barite

Barite's energy serves as a kaleidoscope of the mind. When you are bombarded by a volume of thoughts, this stone quickly reorganizes them all. In this new presentation, clear vivid representations allow you to absorb everything down to the most minute details. The surprising heaviness of this stone anchors you to stay grounded as the mind dissolves confusion with beautiful clarity.
Try this: Journaling Exercise

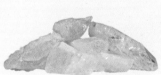

Danburite

Powerful Stone Combinations	Barite + Clear Fluorite
	Danburite + Barite
	Danburite + Amethyst

NERVOUS

The emotional state of nervousness may be daunting. It's the feeling of walking on eggshells with an intimidating force present that prevents us from relaxing or trusting ourselves. We might also ride the edge of nervous excitement, when sensing a big change or shift is about to occur.

Bloodstone

Bloodstone works with nervous energy by processing emotional toxins that may be holding you back or consuming precious energy. It heals the mothering or caretaker wound of losing your identity. When these roles are no longer necessary, a sense of nervousness can occupy the space. Bloodstone's energy helps reclaim power, purpose, and independence, facilitating change.

Try this: Touchstone Practice

Sphalerite

Sphalerite is a wonderful companion for grounding intense nervous energy. It directs any excessive energy to move down through to the lower energy centers of the body as it opens the energetic foot portals to give it an exit. At the same time, it invigorates the creative or sexual energy center.

Try this: Journaling Exercise

Lithium Quartz

Lithium Quartz relieves nervous energy and expels it out of the body. It melts the mind and allows the brain to surrender into the comfort of the heart. It's like a power nap for the soul. It will lay everything down to put the energy to rest. With this stone, you will feel lighter and recalibrated back into positive, clear, and decisive mental health.

Try this: Core Meditation Practice

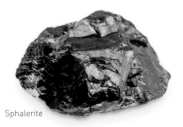

Sphalerite

Powerful Stone Combinations	Black Tourmaline + Lithium Quartz
	Sphalerite + Bloodstone
	Aragonite Star Cluster + Bloodstone

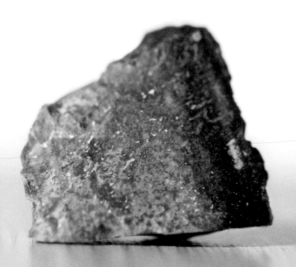

Bloodstone has the ability to
create a protective space in
our emotional field, acting as a
buffer for the nervous system,
allowing us to rest assured in the
present moment.

OVERWHELMED

The experience of overwhelm arises when we have taken on too much at once. The scatterbrained feeling may disconnect us from experiencing a healthy rhythm in everyday life. There may be this constant push and pull of our energy, paired with a dull awareness of the physical or intuitive needs of the self.

Black
Tourmaline

Smoky Quartz

Chrysanthemum
Stone

Sodalite

Sodalite has deeply cleansing abilities to transform overwhelmed energy into a carefree attitude. Its frequency teaches you to trust the process. This stone draws energy out a little at a time, to promote a go-with-the-flow mentality. On a deeper level, Sodalite makes you aware of avoidance behaviors, hesitation, and the roots of the things that lead to overwhelm.
Try this: Sound and Stone Practice

Zoisite

Zoisite is a big confidence booster as it gives you the feeling of having things under control. It helps you prioritize and lends a sense of clarity. The Ruby inclusions often

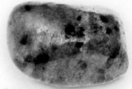

Zoisite

found in Zoisite further amplify its effects by supplying you with the emotional energy needed to handle multiple situations or a high volume of tasks.
Try this: Touchstone Practice

Opal

Opal bears the energy of the emotional nurturer and provides a safe haven to pull yourself together. This stone softens the pieces that are fragmented in order to become whole and balanced. It shines its array of different colors on

energetic debris, clearing it away like a rainbow appearing in the mists of a thunderstorm.
Try this: Conscious Crystal Dreaming

Lapis Lazuli

Lapis Lazuli urges you to come back to peace in the present moment. With its Pyrite inclusions, it allows you to feel grounded in the physical body so the mind does not fly away with itself.
Try this: Movement Meditation

Powerful Stone Combinations

Lapis Lazuli + Smoky Quartz
Sodalite + Zoisite
Opal + Black Tourmaline

ANXIOUS

MORE
CRYSTALS
TO TRY

Anxiety is often rooted in an inability to take action in life, and is usually accompanied by a sense of uneasiness. It can become a huge consumer of our happiness and wellbeing. When we feel anxious, we may also feel vulnerable and at times it may be an instinctive sign that something is not quite right.

Zircon

Amethyst

Galena

Snowflake Obsidian

Snowflake Obsidian is a powerful and protective stone that allows you to release control. When the mind is tailspinning, this stone acts as a peacemaker and will aid you to come back into the body.
Try this: Touchstone Practice

Black Kyanite

Black Kyanite clears the emotional, physical, and mental body in order to

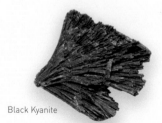

Black Kyanite

become free of constraints. When you feel like a hostage to the mind, this stone will cut the cord that is keeping you imprisoned.
Try this: Core Meditation Practice

Pyrite

Pyrite possesses a primal feeling as ancient as gathering around a fire with its ability to feed life with its reflective light. This stone burns through the negative effects of anxiety as it offers counsel for those who need an outlet to express their wave of fears.
Try this: Journaling Exercise

Red Jasper

Red Jasper opens up your eyes to the root of where the anxiety is stemming from. It offers stability and safety, when you are actively experiencing the anxiety. At this same time, this stone widens your grounding cord to send the palpable anxious energy down into the Earth. Red Jasper coaxes soothing energy to rise back up and move through the body and mind.
Try this: Touchstone Practice

Powerful Stone Combinations

Black Kyanite + Pyrite
Red Jasper + Galena
Snowflake Obsidian + Zircon

IDENTIFYING YOUR EMOTIONS

Kinesthetic reflection

In all the descriptions of emotional and physical states on the previous pages, you may have got clarity on your current emotional climate. If you need more guidance, reflect on these questions to guide you to a specific chapter with emotional themes you may want to explore and further pinpoint if you wish to maintain, enhance, or alter your feelings.

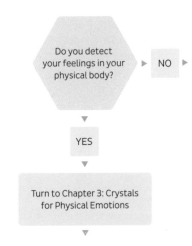

Do you detect your feelings in your physical body?

NO

YES

Turn to Chapter 3: Crystals for Physical Emotions

If yes, does it give you a sense of grounding, expansion, or constriction (do you want to maintain, enhance, or alter)?

Mental reflection

What section did you feel drawn to the most?
Explore the chapter theme indicated there for a list of corresponding emotions.

Crystals for Physical Emotions

Do you feel like you nurture yourself?
Do you feel like you neglect yourself?
Do you feel love easily?
Do you take compliments from others well?
Do you like your body?

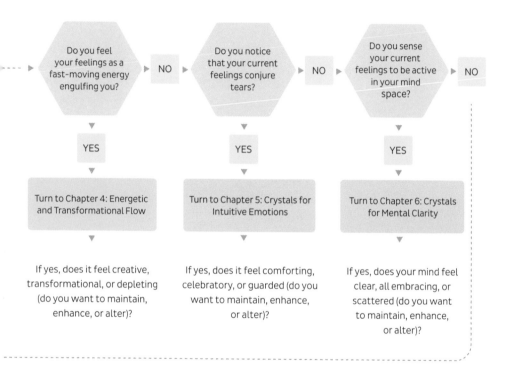

Do you feel your feelings as a fast-moving energy engulfing you? → NO

Do you notice that your current feelings conjure tears? → NO

Do you sense your current feelings to be active in your mind space? → NO

YES

YES

YES

Turn to Chapter 4: Energetic and Transformational Flow

Turn to Chapter 5: Crystals for Intuitive Emotions

Turn to Chapter 6: Crystals for Mental Clarity

If yes, does it feel creative, transformational, or depleting (do you want to maintain, enhance, or alter)?

If yes, does it feel comforting, celebratory, or guarded (do you want to maintain, enhance, or alter)?

If yes, does your mind feel clear, all embracing, or scattered (do you want to maintain, enhance, or alter)?

Energetic and Transformational Flow

Do you have energy all day?
Are you exhausted at any point in your day?
Do you find yourself flaring up?
Are you short-tempered?
Do you hold back your emotions?
Are you confrontational?

Crystals for Intuitive Emotions

Do things in your life seem to flow easily?
Are you stuck in any place in your life?
Do you get discouraged easily?
Do you feel other people's pain?

Crystals for Mental Clarity

Do you feel clear in your thought patterns?
Are you often confused in your day to day life?
Are you a person who worries?
Are you a secure person?
Are you forgetful?

INDEX

ACKNOWLEDGMENTS

Writing this book during a pandemic summoned us to authentically experience each emotional state at a time when the world was also going through a myriad of intensified emotions. With the help of our crystals as tools of emotional support, this book is our positive experience in a collective healing crisis. We are so grateful for the crystals that comprise our personal healing collection of stones. They proved to be steady guides and counsellors and continue to humble and grow us as conscious crystal keepers, time and time again.

A huge heartfelt hug to our beloved Malachi and Meridian, our biggest inspirations. They embody emotional intelligence, showing the potential that can be created by practicing intentional crystal healing from a young age. Their genuine encouragement and shared crystal experiences made this process playful, energetic, and affirming.

A deep thank you to Leo Alberez, who has been our biggest supporter and our strongest teacher throughout the years. Leo has always pushed us to achieve our potential when we didn't see it in ourselves. We love you dearly for believing in us.

To the love of my life, Leah Moon—thank you for always seeing my potential. You are a true gift in my life. You continue to inspire me to be the best version of myself. Your "no" will always feel as good as your "yes".

Thank you to Corynne Alberts for being a spark of creativity when we needed it most. You helped the stone stories come from the heart through uplifting conversations about our collective experiences with them.

A special thank you to Tom Castles, a true artist in the photography studio who graciously allowed us to fill his space with hunks of crystalline earth! It was a delight to play with the crystals together and watch you listen to how they spoke to you.

Our deepest gratitude is to all our clients, healing artists, teachers, classmates, friends, and family who have enriched our lives with their presence. If it wasn't for our community supporting our growth throughout the years, we wouldn't be who we are today.

Lastly, thank you to the universe for linking us together in this wild web of life and giving us the gift of a friendship that has spanned decades. It has been a rock-solid, ever-growing well of infinite love and light that we serve together.

PHOTOGRAPHY CREDITS

Photography by Thomas R. Castles, except the following pages:

Back cover and page 22: Photo by Gabby Conde on Unsplash
Page 1, page 24: Nikki Zalewski/ Shutterstock.com
Page 2, page 9, page 17: ju_see/Shutterstock.com
Page 4: Photo by Rise and co
Page 13: Holly Mazour/Shutterstock.com
Page 15: Photo by Dani Costelo on Unsplash
Page 21: Photo by Kira Auf der Heide on Unsplash
Page 25: Dafinchi/Shutterstock.com
Page 28: olhovyi_photographer/Shutterstock.com
Page 37: photo-world/Shutterstock.com
Page 45: Lephototo/Shutterstock.com

Page 55, page 113: olhovyi_photographer/Shutterstock.com
Page 67: Roy Palmer/Shutterstock.com
Page 71: pukka luna/Shutterstock.com
Page 75: Collective Arcana/Shutterstock.com
Page 81: Photo by Rise and co
Page 85: SageElyse/Shutterstock.com
Page 87: Minakryn Ruslan/Shutterstock.com
Page 99: Photo by Benjamin Lehman on Unsplash
Page 103: tanya_morozz/Shutterstock.com
Page 107: Stellar Gems/Shutterstock.com